HEALTH CARE IN TRANSITION

HEALTH CARE CONSOLIDATION UNDER THE AFFORDABLE CARE ACT

HEALTH CARE IN TRANSITION

Additional books and e-books in this series can be found on Nova's website under the Series tab.

HEALTH CARE IN TRANSITION

HEALTH CARE CONSOLIDATION UNDER THE AFFORDABLE CARE ACT

DOMINIK VOGEL
EDITOR

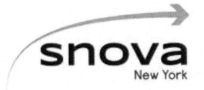

Copyright © 2019 by Nova Science Publishers, Inc.

All rights reserved. No part of this book may be reproduced, stored in a retrieval system or transmitted in any form or by any means: electronic, electrostatic, magnetic, tape, mechanical photocopying, recording or otherwise without the written permission of the Publisher.

We have partnered with Copyright Clearance Center to make it easy for you to obtain permissions to reuse content from this publication. Simply navigate to this publication's page on Nova's website and locate the "Get Permission" button below the title description. This button is linked directly to the title's permission page on copyright.com. Alternatively, you can visit copyright.com and search by title, ISBN, or ISSN.

For further questions about using the service on copyright.com, please contact:
Copyright Clearance Center
Phone: +1-(978) 750-8400   Fax: +1-(978) 750-4470   E-mail: info@copyright.com.

NOTICE TO THE READER

The Publisher has taken reasonable care in the preparation of this book, but makes no expressed or implied warranty of any kind and assumes no responsibility for any errors or omissions. No liability is assumed for incidental or consequential damages in connection with or arising out of information contained in this book. The Publisher shall not be liable for any special, consequential, or exemplary damages resulting, in whole or in part, from the readers' use of, or reliance upon, this material. Any parts of this book based on government reports are so indicated and copyright is claimed for those parts to the extent applicable to compilations of such works.

Independent verification should be sought for any data, advice or recommendations contained in this book. In addition, no responsibility is assumed by the Publisher for any injury and/or damage to persons or property arising from any methods, products, instructions, ideas or otherwise contained in this publication.

This publication is designed to provide accurate and authoritative information with regard to the subject matter covered herein. It is sold with the clear understanding that the Publisher is not engaged in rendering legal or any other professional services. If legal or any other expert assistance is required, the services of a competent person should be sought. FROM A DECLARATION OF PARTICIPANTS JOINTLY ADOPTED BY A COMMITTEE OF THE AMERICAN BAR ASSOCIATION AND A COMMITTEE OF PUBLISHERS.

Additional color graphics may be available in the e-book version of this book.

Library of Congress Cataloging-in-Publication Data

ISBN: 978-1-53616-870-9

Published by Nova Science Publishers, Inc. † New York

CONTENTS

Preface		vii
Chapter 1	Examining the Impact of Healthcare Consolidation	1
Chapter 2	Examining the Effectiveness of the Individual Mandate under the Affordable Care Act	181
Index		259
Related Nova Publications		271

PREFACE

When the Affordable Care Act was just beginning to be implemented in 2013, the HHS secretary released a report stating the goal of Affordable Healthcare Act is to increase competition and transparency in the markets for individuals and small group insurance leading to higher quality, more affordable products. Fast forward 4 years later, what we are seeing is a decrease in competition and an increase in premium costs. This trend is concerning for all Americans and is discussed in this book.

In: Health Care Consolidation ...
Editor: Dominik Vogel
ISBN: 978-1-53616-870-9
© 2019 Nova Science Publishers, Inc.

Chapter 1

EXAMINING THE IMPACT OF HEALTHCARE CONSOLIDATION*

WEDNESDAY, FEBRUARY 14, 2018

HOUSE OF REPRESENTATIVES, SUBCOMMITTEE ON
OVERSIGHT AND INVESTIGATIONS, COMMITTEE ON ENERGY
AND COMMERCE,
Washington, DC.

The subcommittee met, pursuant to call, at 10:17 a.m., in room 2322, Rayburn House Office Building, Hon. Gregg Harper (chairman of the subcommittee) presiding.

Members present: Representatives Harper, Griffith, Burgess, Brooks, Collins, Barton, Walberg, Walters, Costello, Carter, Walden (ex officio), DeGette, Schakowsky, Castor, Tonko, Ruiz, Peters, and Pallone (ex officio).

---

* This is an edited, reformatted and augmented version of Hearing before the Subcommittee on Oversight and Investigations of the Committee on Energy and Commerce, House of Representatives, One Hundred Fifteenth Congress, Second Session, Publication No. Serial No. 115–99, dated February 14, 2018.

Staff present: Jennifer Barblan, Chief Counsel, Oversight and Investigations; Adam Buckalew, Professional Staff Member, Health; Zack Dareshori, Legislative Clerk; Lamar Echols, Counsel, Oversight and Investigations; Margaret Tucker Fogarty, Staff Assistant; Ed Kim, Policy Coordinator, Health; Jennifer Sherman, Press Secretary; Natalie Turner, Counsel, Oversight and Investigations; Hamlin Wade, Special Advisor for External Affairs; Jeff Carroll, Minority Staff Director; Evan Gilbert, Minority Press Assistant; Tiffany Guarascio, Minority Deputy Staff Director and Chief Health Advisor; Zach Kahan, Minority Outreach and Member Services Coordinator; Christopher Knauer, Minority Oversight Staff Director; Miles Lichtman, Minority Policy Analyst; Kevin McAloon, Minority Professional Staff Member; Andrew Souvall, Minority Director of Communications, Outreach and Member Services; and C.J. Young, Minority Press Secretary.

Mr. Harper. The subcommittee convenes this hearing entitled "Examining the Impact of Healthcare Consolidation."

I want to welcome our witnesses, who will be introduced in more detail momentarily. The Chair will now recognize himself for purposes of an opening statement.

OPENING STATEMENT OF HON. GREGG HARPER, A REPRESENTATIVE IN CONGRESS FROM THE STATE OF MISSISSIPPI

The price of healthcare in the United States has steadily risen for several decades. In 2016, U.S. healthcare spending was estimated to be around $3.3 trillion, and the gross domestic product related to healthcare spending was 17.9 percent, an increase from 17.7 percent just the year before.

Data shows that the increasing costs of healthcare are ultimately passed along to American workers and families. This trend is concerning for all Americans and is an issue the committee will continue to examine here today and in the future.

While there are numerous factors contributing to the rising cost of healthcare, reports and studies show consolidation is a contributing factor.

Consolidation is not a new phenomenon. It has been occurring for decades among hospitals, doctors, the pharmaceutical industry, and insurance companies.

To date, most studies and data have focused on hospital and insurer consolidations. The effects of cross-market consolidations and other types of vertical consolidations are less clear.

Horizontal hospital consolidation—the consolidation of hospitals into a single larger system—has grown at a rapid pace this past decade.

According to the Medicare Payment Advisory Commission, MedPAC, hospital markets are now highly consolidated. In 2012, MedPAC found that a single hospital system counted for a majority of Medicare discharges in 146 of 391 metropolitan areas.

Similarly, a researcher found that in 2016, 90 percent of metropolitan areas were highly concentrated for hospitals. Through vertical consolidation, hospitals have also acquired a significant number of physician practices over the past decade.

A recent analysis shows that the number of physicians employed by hospitals increased by 49 percent between 2012 and 2015. The Government Accountability Office found that between 2007 to 2014 the number of vertically consolidated physicians nearly doubled, from 9,600 to 182,000.

There also appears to be a significant amount of consolidation in the health insurance industry. The estimated nationwide market share of largest four insurers increased from 74 percent in 2006 to 83 percent in 2014.

Recently, the U.S. Department of Justice successfully blocked two mergers between major health insurance companies, noting that the mergers would violate antitrust laws and would lead to higher healthcare costs for consumers.

Given DOJ's success in challenging these mergers, some analysts have speculated that we will start seeing more vertical integration in the healthcare space.

Additionally, the FTC—Federal Trade Commission—has recently been successful challenging horizontal mergers of providers that supply similar services in geographic proximity.

However, the FTC and DOJ do not appear to regularly challenge vertical consolidations. Since 2000, the FTC and DOJ have challenged only 22 total vertical mergers.

The move towards consolidation raises questions as to what is really meant and what this really means for patients. Hospitals and providers contend that consolidation makes facilities more efficient by eliminating duplicative services, reducing administrative burdens, and improving quality of care.

Physicians are incentivized for many reasons to consolidate with hospitals, including more payment stability and less financial and regulatory burdens.

Many experts point to Medicare paying more for the same services at hospitals than at a physician's office as a leading factor in providers consolidating with hospitals.

While many benefits of consolidation are difficult to measure, the majority of studies and literature shows that horizontal hospital consolidation leads to higher prices.

For example, according to MedPAC, horizontal consolidation of hospitals has contributed to the discrepancy between prices Medicare pays hospitals and what commercial insurers pay.

In fact, a study found that in 2012, the average private price was 75 percent higher than Medicare prices after hospitals consolidate. Additionally, a 2018 study looked at hospital and physician consolidations. It found that from 2007 to 2013 almost 10 percent of physician practices reviewed were acquired by a hospital.

After being acquired, the services offered by physicians increased an average of 14 percent. In response to the growing number of consolidations in the healthcare industry, in October of 2017, the Trump administration issued an executive order to foster greater competition in the healthcare markets and directing the administration to promote competition in and limit excessive consolidation in the healthcare system.

Health and Human Services was directed to collect public comments on these issues, and we look forward to hearing and learning what innovative solutions HHS discovers during this process.

Consolidation in the healthcare industry raises many important questions relating to competition and innovation. For instance: Why has consolidation increased during the past decade? Is consolidation good for patients? What changes could Congress or HHS make to encourage competition and innovation in healthcare?

I welcome and thank the witnesses for being here. We look forward to their testimony.

[The prepared statement of Mr. Harper follows:]

PREPARED STATEMENT OF HON. GREGG HARPER

The subcommittee convenes this hearing entitled "Examining the Impact of Healthcare Consolidation."

The price of healthcare in the United States has steadily risen for several decades. In 2016, U.S. healthcare spending was estimated to be around $3.3 trillion, and the gross domestic product related to healthcare spending was 17.9 percent, an increase from 17.7 percent just the year before. Data shows that the increasing costs of healthcare are ultimately passed along to American workers and families. This trend is concerning for all Americans and is an issue the committee will continue to examine here today and in the future.

While there are numerous factors contributing to the rising costs of healthcare, reports and studies show consolidation is a contributing factor. Consolidation is not a new phenomenon. It has been occurring for decades among hospitals, doctors, the pharmaceutical industry, and insurance companies.

To date, most studies and data have focused on hospital and insurer consolidations. The effects of cross-market consolidations and other types of vertical consolidations are less clear.

Horizontal hospital consolidation—the consolidation of hospitals into a single larger system—has grown at a rapid pace the past decade. According to the Medicare Payment Advisory Commission (MedPAC), hospital markets are now highly consolidated. In 2012, MedPAC found that a single hospital system accounted for a majority of Medicare discharges in 146 of 391 metropolitan areas. Similarly, a researcher found that in 2016, 90 percent of metropolitan areas were highly concentrated for hospitals.

Through vertical consolidation, hospitals have also acquired a significant number of physician practices over the past decade. A recent analysis shows that the number of physicians employed by hospitals increased by 49 percent between 2012 and 2015.

The Government Accountability Office found that between 2007 to 2014, the number of vertically consolidated physicians nearly doubled from about 96,000 to 182,000.

There also appears to be a significant amount of consolidation in the health insurance industry. The estimated nationwide market share of the largest four insurers increased from 74 percent in 2006 to 83 percent in 2014. Recently, the U.S. Department of Justice (DOJ) successfully blocked two mergers between major health insurance companies, noting that the mergers would violate antitrust laws and would lead to higher healthcare costs for consumers.

Given DOJ's success in challenging these mergers, some analysts have speculated that we'll start seeing more vertical integration in the healthcare space. Additionally, the Federal Trade Commission (FTC) has recently been successful challenging horizontal mergers of providers that supply similar services in geographic proximity.

However, the FTC and DOJ do not appear to regularly challenge vertical consolidations. Since 2000, the FTC and DOJ have challenged only 22 vertical mergers in total.

The move toward consolidation raises questions as to what it really means for patients. Hospitals and providers contend that consolidation makes facilities more efficient by eliminating duplicative services, reducing administrative burdens, and improving quality of care. Physicians are incentivized for many reasons to consolidate with hospitals, including more payment stability and less financial and regulatory burdens. Many experts point to Medicare paying more for the same services at hospitals than a physician's office as a leading factor in providers consolidating with hospitals.

While many benefits of consolidation are difficult to measure, the majority of studies and literature shows that horizontal hospital consolidation leads to higher prices.

For example, according to MedPAC, horizontal consolidation of hospitals has contributed to the discrepancy between prices Medicare pays hospitals and what commercial insurers pay. In fact, a study found that in 2012, the average private price was 75 percent higher than Medicare prices after hospitals consolidate. Additionally, a 2018 study looking at hospital/physician consolidations found that from 2007 to 2013, almost 10 percent of physician practices reviewed were acquired by a hospital. After being acquired, the services offered by physicians increased an average of 14 percent.

In response to the growing number of consolidations in the healthcare industry, in October 2017, the Trump administration issued an Executive Order to foster greater competition in the healthcare markets and directing the administration to promote competition in and limit excessive consolidation in the healthcare system. Health and Human Services was directed to collect public comments on these issues.

We look forward to learning what innovative solutions HHS discovers during this process.

Consolidation in the healthcare industry raises many important questions relating to competition and innovation.

- Why has consolidation increased during the past decade?
- Is consolidation good for patients?

- What changes could Congress or HHS make to encourage competition and innovation in healthcare?

I welcome and thank the witnesses, and look forward to their testimony.

Mr. HARPER. At this time, the Chair will recognize the ranking member of the subcommittee, Ms. DeGette.

OPENING STATEMENT OF HON. DIANA DEGETTE, A REPRESENTATIVE IN CONGRESS FROM THE STATE OF COLORADO

Ms. DEGETTE. Thank you so much, Mr. Chairman.

As we will hear from the witnesses today, we have seen a long-term trend in consolidation in the healthcare sector, where the market has become increasingly dominated by fewer and fewer companies.

This trend goes back 20 years or more and, frankly, it had real impacts on consumers. Excessive consolidation leaves consumers with few choices, which not only limits their care options but also has the potential to raise prices.

And it's not just individual consumers who are paying more. When Medicare's expenditures go up, then taxpayers suffer as well.

You know, it's important to note consolidation is not per se negative. Hospital mergers can enable providers to combine resources and improve coordination of care.

But, if increased market power allows them to raise their prices with no competitive alternatives, then entire communities can suffer.

We have also seen increasing numbers of hospitals acquiring physician practices. Twenty Sixteen marked the first time that less than half of physicians own their own practice. Again, this can result in increased expenditures when the same services are now provided but at higher prices.

Although hospitals point to the reduced inefficiencies and regulatory burdens on physicians that can result from these acquisitions, it's really clear that the delivery of care is changing, and not always to the benefit of patients and payers.

Likewise, when insurance companies are able to pull their market power to negotiate lower rates, there can be positive results. But not so when they push the other competitors out of the market or when the savings are not passed on to consumers.

For example, last year we saw the courts strike down two mergers between large insurers. These companies were already among the biggest players in the market, and it was recognized that the merged companies would stifle competition and innovation.

It's really possible that we're going to see more attempted mergers of this kind, and consumers need to get advocates on their behalf.

These issues affect all segments of the healthcare market, including prescription drugs. As you know, Mr. Chairman, I've long been concerned about the rising price of drugs, and insulin in particular.

Congressman Tom Reed and I were the co-chairs of the Diabetes Caucus, and we are in the process of conducting an inquiry into insulin prices.

Our early findings suggest that consolidation across different parts of the so-called drug supply chain is indeed affecting what patients pay for their medications.

The problem has ramifications not just for consumers who rely on these medicines but also for the employers and public and private insurance companies that pay for them.

And, so as we talk about these issues, it's important to know that pharmacy benefit managers have also seen this sort of consolidation we are going to hear about today.

PBMs have an enormous influence in the prescription drug market, and yet the entire market is dominated by just a few of them.

So I am eager to hear the witnesses' thoughts on these issues. It's going to be my line of questioning, so you can start to think about that now and what we can do to address it.

Frankly, we also need more innovative solutions that have potential to upend the inefficiencies in the market. Amazon, J.P. Morgan, and Berkshire Hathaway recently made news when they announced a joint venture to reduce healthcare costs for their companies.

Well, it remains to be seen how effective this merger will be, but it does show that there is a need in the market for innovation.

Mr. Chairman, these are complex issues and we're not going to solve them today, even with our best efforts. While I recognize there can be legitimate and even good reasons for consolidation, the long-term trends are alarming, and the need for new approaches is clear.

I look forward to hearing from the witnesses about what the research tells us are these underlying problems, what the real-world effects are, and what we can do to help.

And with that, I yield back.

[The prepared statement of Ms. DeGette follows:]

PREPARED STATEMENT OF HON. DIANA DEGETTE

Thank you, Mr. Chairman. As we will hear from the witnesses today, we have seen a long-term trend in consolidation in the healthcare sector, where the market has become increasing dominated by fewer companies. This trend goes back 20 years or more, and it has real effects on all consumers.

Excessive consolidation leaves consumers with few choices, which not only limits their care options, but can also raise their prices. And let's not forget that it is not just individual consumers who are paying more: when Medicare's expenditures go up, the taxpayers suffer as well.

Consolidation does not always have to be negative. Hospital mergers can enable providers to combine their resources and improve coordination of care. But if their increased market power allows them to raise their prices with no alternative for consumers, entire communities can suffer.

We have also seen increasing numbers of hospitals acquiring physician practices. Twenty Sixteen marked the first time that less than half of physicians owned their own practice. This can result in increased expenditures when the same services are now paid at higher rates. Although hospitals point to the reduced inefficiencies and regulatory burdens on physicians that result from these acquisitions, it is clear that the delivery of care is changing, and not always to the benefit of patients and payers.

Likewise, when insurance companies are able to pool their market power to negotiate lower rates, there can be positive results—but not when they push all other competitors out of the market, or when the savings are not passed down to consumers.

For instance, a year ago we saw the courts strike down two mergers between large insurers. These companies were already among the biggest players in the market, and it was recognized that the merged companies would stifle competition and innovation. It is very possible we will see more attempted mergers of this kind, and consumers need advocates on their behalf.

These issues affect all segments of the healthcare market, including prescription drugs. As you know, Mr. Chairman, I have long been concerned about the rising price of drugs, and insulin in particular. Congressman Tom Reed (R–NY) and I are in the process of conducting an inquiry into insulin prices through the Diabetes Caucus. Our early findings suggest that consolidation across different parts of the so-called "drug supply chain" is indeed affecting what patients pay for their medicines. This problem has ramifications not just for the consumers who rely on these medicines, but also the employers and private and public insurance programs that pay for them.

So as we talk about these issues, it is important to note that pharmacy benefit managers (PBMs) have also seen the sort of consolidation we will hear about today. PBMs have enormous influence in the prescription drug market, and yet the entire market is dominated by just a few PBMs. I am eager to hear the witnesses' thoughts on this problem, and what more can be done to address it.

We also need more innovative solutions that have potential to upend the inefficiencies in the market. Amazon, J.P. Morgan, and Berkshire

Hathaway recently made news when they announced a joint venture to reduce healthcare costs for their companies. While it remains to be seen how effective this venture will be, it clearly shows there is a need in the market for innovation.

Mr. Chairman, these are complex issues, and the solutions will not be simple. While I recognize that there can be legitimate and even beneficial reasons for consolidation, the long-term trends are alarming, and the need for new approaches is clear. I look forward to hearing from the witnesses about what the research tells us are the underlying problems, what the real-word effects are, and what steps we can take to help.

I yield back.

Mr. HARPER. The gentlewoman yields back.
The Chair will now recognize the chairman of the full committee, Mr. Walden, for purposes of an opening statement.

OPENING STATEMENT OF HON. GREG WALDEN, A REPRESENTATIVE IN CONGRESS FROM THE STATE OF OREGON

Mr. WALDEN. Well, thank you, Chairman Harper. We appreciate your leadership on these issues.

As you mentioned in your opening statement, healthcare costs continue to rise in the United States. We are all paying higher costs.

In 2016 alone, the U.S. spent about $3.3 trillion—that's more than $10,000 per person—on healthcare. And as I've said on numerous occasions, this committee is dedicated to investigating all of the cost drivers in our healthcare system from top to bottom.

For example, we have been looking at the 340B drug pricing program for the past 2 years, and just last month we issued our report. Pretty comprehensive on the findings and recommendations.

Last December, the Health Subcommittee held a hearing examining the drug supply chain and the impact each participant's supply chain has and the ultimate cost to patients.

And today we want to explore consolidation in the healthcare industry and the impact consolidation has on consumers. Mergers and acquisitions are changing the healthcare landscape across the United States and over the past few years there is been a continuous stream of horizontal and vertical merger announcements between hospitals, insurers, physician groups, pharmaceutical companies, pharmaceutical benefit managers, pharmacies, and other healthcare firms, and those are just the deals we know about.

Some mergers are so small they don't make it onto the congressional radar screen, and in the aggregate, however, even these small mergers could have an impact on consumers—sometimes positively, sometimes negatively.

So one of the central questions that I hope we explore today is, What does this consolidation mean for patients? My principle is: Put the consumers first and you'll have pretty good policy, because that means you've got competition, drives innovation and choice, and should drive down price.

On the one hand, consolidation is potentially good for patients by reducing the cost of care and improving outcomes through improved efficiencies and better care coordination. It can be that.

On the other hand, we are concerned that some consolidation could actually lead to higher prices for patients, doesn't lead to improved quality of care, and so we want to hear both perspectives today and what the right public policy position should be.

So today, we also want to explore how consolidation impacts innovation. Last month, we all heard the news that Amazon, Berkshire Hathaway, and J.P. Morgan are going to partner, try to improve employee satisfaction, reduce healthcare costs for their United States employees.

That sure caught my attention because, if you want to talk about disruptors, I think at least Amazon you'd put at the top of the list of how to disrupt things that are otherwise bureaucratically constrained. And with the horsepower of Berkshire Hathaway and J.P. Morgan, something big could happen in this space, and it needs to.

Although we still know very little about their plans, I am intrigued by this partnership, and we will continue to monitor it closely, and when they are ready to come share information with us, we will be all open arms to hear how it's going to work.

Similarly, a group of several hospital systems recently announced their decision to enter the generic drug industry and develop a not-for-profit generic drug company. One thing I'd like to hear more about today is whether consolidation makes it more or less likely that we will see innovation in the healthcare market.

And finally, we also need a better understanding of what's driving consolidation, whether Congress should be trying to do anything about it.

We have heard a lot about how disparities in payments across sites of service may result in market consolidation, and as a result Congress took a step toward equalizing payment rates across different sites of care through the Bipartisan Budget Act of 2015.

But we continue to hear about some of these inequities in payment rates. And as I mentioned earlier, the committee has been closely examining the 340B program. During this work, we found 340B program creates an incentive for hospitals to acquire independent physician offices that are not eligible for 340B discounts, especially in the oncology space.

One report showed there was a 172 percent increase in the consolidation of community oncology practices since 2008. A recent article in the New England Journal of Medicine found, among other things, that the 340B program has been associated with hospital consolidation in hematology oncology.

So as evidenced by these examples, the committee needs to carefully review these types of policies and ensure that any Federal policies that create incentives for consolidation are appropriate and ultimately benefit patients and consumers.

[The prepared statement of Mr. Walden follows:]

PREPARED STATEMENT OF HON. GREG WALDEN

Thank you, Mr. Chairman, for holding this hearing on the very important issue of consolidation in the healthcare industry.

As Chairman Harper mentioned in his opening statement, healthcare costs continue to rise in the United States. In 2016 alone, the U.S. spent about $3.3 trillion-more than $10,000 per person-on healthcare.

As I've said on numerous occasions, this committee is dedicated to investigating the cost drivers in our healthcare system from top to bottom.

For example, we have been looking into the 340B Drug Pricing Program for the past 2 years. Just last month, the committee issued a comprehensive report detailing its 340B investigation and findings. Last December, the Health Subcommittee held a hearing examining the drug supply chain and the impact each participant in the supply chain has in the ultimate cost to patients.

Today we want to explore consolidation in the healthcare industry and the impact of consolidation on consumers.

Mergers and acquisitions are changing the healthcare landscape across the country. Over the past few years, there has been a continuous stream of horizontal and vertical merger announcements between hospitals, insurers, physician groups, pharmaceutical companies, pharmaceutical benefit managers, pharmacies, and other healthcare firms. And those are just the deals we know about-some mergers are so small they don't make it onto our radar. In the aggregate, however, even these small mergers may have an impact on consumers.

One of the central questions that we want to explore today is what does this consolidation mean for patients? On the one hand, consolidation is potentially good for patients by reducing the cost of care and improving outcomes through improved efficiencies and better care coordination. On the other hand, we're concerned that some consolidation could lead to higher prices for patients and not improve the quality of care that they receive from their doctor. I look forward to hearing more on both perspectives from our witnesses today.

Today we also want to explore how consolidation impacts innovation. Last month, we all heard the news that Amazon, Berkshire Hathaway, and JP Morgan are going to partner and try to improve employee satisfaction and reduce healthcare costs for their U.S. employees. Although we still know very little about their plans, I'm intrigued by this partnership and plan to continue to closely monitor it as the plans develop. Similarly, a group of several hospital systems recently announced their decision to enter the generic drug industry and develop a not-for-profit generic drug company. One thing I'd like to hear more about today is whether consolidation makes it more-or less-likely that we will see innovation in the healthcare market.

Finally, we also need to better understand what is driving consolidation and whether Congress should be trying to do anything about it.

We've heard a lot about how disparities in payments across sites of service may result in market consolidation, and as a result, Congress took a step toward equalizing payments rates across different sites of care through the Bipartisan Budget Act of 2015. We continue to hear concerns about inequities in payment rates.

As I previously mentioned, the committee has been closely examining the 340B program over the past 2 years. During this work, we found that the 340B program creates an incentive for hospitals to acquire independent physician offices that are not eligible for the 340B discount-especially in the oncology space. One report showed that there was a 172 percent increase in the consolidation of community oncology practices since 2008. A recent article in the New England Journal of Medicine found among other things that the 340B program has been associated with hospital consolidation in hematology-oncology.

As evidenced by these examples, the committee needs to carefully review these types of policies and ensure that any Federal policies that create incentives for consolidation are appropriate and ultimately benefit patients and consumers.

I would like to thank the witnesses for testifying here today and I look forward to hearing your testimony.

Mr. WALDEN. I now yield to Dr. Burgess the remainder of my time.

Mr. BURGESS. Well, thank you, Mr. Chairman, and I want to take a moment to acknowledge that one of our witnesses this morning, Dr. Dafny, is the daughter of Nachum Dafny, who taught me neuroscience a long time ago at the University of Texas Medical School at Houston, affectionately known by the acronym "UTMUSH" by its friends. But I understand Dr. Dafny is still active in teaching, and so I was grateful to learn that this morning and certainly want to welcome Dr. Dafny to our subcommittee.

Mr. Chairman, I also have a unanimous consent request. It's probably just an oversight that we don't have a witness here talking about physician ownership of facilities.

So I have a paper from Health Affairs. It was published March of 2008, and, while that was 10 years ago, it does not diminish the overall brilliance and the keen insights provided in this paper, and it was actually written by your humble chairman of the Health Subcommittee.

So I ask unanimous consent to put that into the record. Mr. HARPER. Without objection.

[The information appears at the conclusion of the hearing.]

Ms. DEGETTE. Wait a minute. I am going to have to reserve——

[Laughter.]

Ms. DEGETTE. I am going to reserve a point of order on that.

Mr. HARPER. It was questionable, but without objection, it is admitted.

With that, the Chair will now recognize Mr. Pallone, the ranking member of the full committee, for the purposes of an opening statement.

OPENING STATEMENT OF HON. FRANK PALLONE, JR., A REPRESENTATIVE IN CONGRESS FROM THE STATE OF NEW JERSEY

Mr. PALLONE. Thank you, Mr. Chairman.

The issues we will hear about today are critical for understanding the healthcare market. We have continued to see a long-term trend of consolidation in the healthcare industry, including among providers and insurers, and it's important we look at these trends with careful scrutiny.

While consolidation is not necessarily a bad thing, it's important we understand the implications for consumers. I often worry, Mr. Chairman, that the people who do the consolidation want to say that it's great and rosy and they do, you know, put out all kinds of propaganda and literature and billboards saying how great it is, but that doesn't necessarily mean it's the case.

For example, when insurance companies merge they often cite the advantages of increased market power to reduce administrative costs and negotiate lower prices. However, that has not always been the result. In fact, research has shown that some insurer mergers have led to increased premiums for consumers, and this is something we need to be watching very closely.

If the insurance market becomes dominated by fewer companies that only grow bigger, consumers will not benefit. For example, in 2016 the Department of Justice had to intervene in Aetna's acquisition of Humana as well as Anthem's acquisition of Cigna.

The courts determined that those deals would have hurt competition and innovation, and 1 year ago today the two mergers were called off.

Although those mergers were canceled, these trends are continuing and have been building for quite some time. Fifteen years ago, most States saw a third of their market controlled by a single insurer.

That consolidation continues to accelerate to the point where in 2014 the top four insurers controlled 83 percent of the market nationwide.

More recently, CVS Health announced that it would acquire the insurer Aetna. While it's still too early to tell what this merger will mean for consumers, it certainly raises questions about how competitive the market will be and how these types of vertical consolidations will affect the delivery of care.

Instead of the market being dominated by a few large companies, it's important for consumers to have choices when picking their insurance plans. This insures not only a wider array of health benefits to fit their needs, but also brings down consumer costs.

For instance, the Department of Health and Human Services found that higher numbers of insurers were associated with slow growth in insurance premiums.

Providers have also not been immune to these consolidation trends. Between '98 and 2015, there were over 1,400 hospital mergers and acquisitions. Certainly, that's the case in my State of New Jersey. In 2015, the number of hospitals involved in such deals was more than three times what it was in 2008.

Now, some consolidation in the market may be inevitable. But, just as we critically examine insurance mergers with an eye to the impact on consumers, our first concern with provider consolidation should also be with the patients who will be affected.

Hospitals often point to the advantages of consolidation, such as reduced costs of capital and benefits of scale. However, we have also seen some evidence that mergers can lead to increased prices for hospital care. The GAO has found that it's also true in vertical consolidations. When hospitals acquire physician practices, Medicare expenditures can go up as care is provided in more expensive hospital outpatient settings.

And prices should not be our only concern. While a larger hospital system may be able to provide more services, it's not at all clear that provider consolidation necessarily leads to better quality of care.

So these are complex issues, and I look forward to hearing what the latest research says about the long-term trends in consolidation and, most importantly, what the effects are for consumers.

And unless one of my colleagues wants the time, I'll yield back, Mr. Chairman.

[The prepared statement of Mr. Pallone follows:]

PREPARED STATEMENT OF HON. FRANK PALLONE, JR.

The issues we will hear about today are critical for understanding the healthcare market. We have continued to see a long-term trend of consolidation in the healthcare industry, including among providers and insurers—and it is important we look at these trends with careful scrutiny.

While consolidation is not necessarily a bad thing in all instances, it is important we understand the implications for consumers.

For example, when insurance companies merge, they often cite the advantages of increased market power to reduce administrative costs and negotiate lower prices. However, that has not always been the result. In fact, research has shown that some insurer mergers have led to increased premiums for consumers. This is something we need to be watching very closely.

If the insurance market becomes dominated by fewer companies that only grow bigger, consumers will not benefit. For example, in 2016, the Department of Justice had to intervene in Aetna's acquisition of Humana, as well as Anthem's acquisition of Cigna. The courts determined that those deals would have hurt competition and innovation, and 1 year ago today, the two mergers were called off.

Although those mergers were canceled, these trends are continuing, and have been building for quite some time. Fifteen years ago, most States saw a third of their market controlled by a single insurer. That consolidation continues to accelerate to the point where in 2014, the top four insurers controlled 83 percent of the market nationwide.

More recently, CVS Health announced that it would acquire the insurer Aetna. While it is still too early to tell what this merger will mean for consumers, it certainly raises questions about how competitive the market will be and how these types of vertical consolidations will affect the delivery of care.

Instead of the market being dominated by a few large companies, it is important for consumers to have choices when picking their insurance plans. This ensures not only a wider array of health benefits to fit their needs, but also helps bring down consumer costs. For instance, the

Department of Health and Human Services found that higher numbers of insurers were associated with slowed growth in insurance premiums.

Providers have also not been immune to these consolidation trends. Between 1998 and 2015 there were over 1,400 hospital mergers and acquisitions. In 2015, the number of hospitals involved in such deals was more than three times what it was in 2008.

Now, some consolidation in the market may be inevitable. But just as we critically examine insurer mergers with an eye on the impact on consumers, our first concern with provider consolidation should also be with the patients who will be affected.

Hospitals often point to advantages of consolidation, such as reduced costs of capital and benefits of scale. However, we have also seen some evidence that mergers can lead to increased prices for hospital care.

The Government Accountability Office has found that this is also true in vertical consolidations: when hospitals acquire physician practices, Medicare expenditures can go up as care is provided in more expensive hospital outpatient settings.

And prices should not be our only concern here. While a larger hospital system may be able to provide more services, it is not clear that provider consolidation necessarily leads to better quality of care.

These are complex issues, and I look forward to hearing what the latest research says about the long-term trends in consolidation, and most importantly, what the effects are for consumers.

Thank you, I yield back.

Mr. HARPER. The gentleman yields back.

I ask unanimous consent that the Members' written opening statements be made part of the record, and without objection they will so be entered into the record.

I would now like to introduce our panel of witnesses for today's hearing. Today we have Dr. Martin Gaynor, the E.J. Barone University professor of economics and health policy at Carnegie Mellon University. Welcome, sir. We are glad to have you with us today.

Next is Leemore Dafny. Dr. Leemore Dafny, who is the Bruce V. Rauner professor of business administration at Harvard Business School. Welcome, Dr. Dafny. We are honored to have you with us.

And finally, Dr. Kevin Schulman, professor of medicine, visiting scholar at Harvard Business School, and associate director of the Duke Clinical Research Institute. We welcome you as well.

I want to thank each of you for being here, providing testimony to us and insight into this important topic, and we look forward to the opportunity to discuss healthcare consolidation today.

And I know that you're aware that the committee is holding an investigative hearing, and when so doing we have the practice of taking testimony under oath.

Do any of you have an objection to testifying under oath?

Seeing none, the Chair then advises you that under the rules of the House and the rules of the committee, you are entitled to be accompanied by counsel.

Do you desire to be accompanied by counsel during your testimony today?

Everyone has responded in the negative.

In that case, if you would please rise, raise your right hand, and I will swear you in.

[Witnesses sworn.]

Thank you. They all have responded affirmatively, and thank you for that. You're now under oath and subject to the penalties set forth in Title 18, Section 1001 of the United States Code, and you may now give a 5-minute summary of your written testimony.

And at this point, I will recognize Dr. Gaynor first for the purpose of his opening statement.

Sir, you have 5 minutes.

STATEMENTS OF MARTIN GAYNOR, PH.D., E.J. BARONE UNIVERSITY PROFESSOR OF ECONOMICS AND HEALTH POLICY, HEINZ COLLEGE, CARNEGIE MELLON UNIVERSITY; LEEMORE S. DAFNY, PH.D., BRUCE V. RAUNER PROFESSOR OF BUSINESS ADMINISTRATION, HARVARD BUSINESS SCHOOL; AND KEVIN A. SCHULMAN, M.D., PROFESSOR OF MEDICINE, DUKE UNIVERSITY, AND VISITING SCHOLAR, HARVARD BUSINESS SCHOOL

Statement of Martin Gaynor

Dr. GAYNOR. Thank you.
Chairman Harper, Ranking Member DeGette, members of the subcommittee and the committee, thank you for holding a hearing on this vitally important topic and for giving me the opportunity to testify in front of you today.

I am an economist who has been studying the healthcare sector and specifically healthcare markets and competition for nearly 40 years. I am the E.J. Barone University professor of economics and public policy at the Heinz College of Public Policy at Carnegie Mellon University in Pittsburgh, Pennsylvania.

I served as the director of the Bureau of Economics of the Federal Trade Commission in 2013 and 2014, during which time I was involved in the many healthcare matters that came before the commission.

I've also served the Commonwealth of Pennsylvania as a member of the Governor's Healthcare Advisory Board and as co-chair of its working group on shoppable healthcare.

The U.S. healthcare system is based on markets. The system will work only as well as the markets that underpin it. These markets do not function as well as they could or should.

Prices are high and rising. They're incomprehensible and egregious— pricing practices. Quality is suboptimal, and the sector is sluggish and unresponsive, in contrast to the innovation and dynamism which characterize much of the rest of our economy. Lack of competition has a lot to do with these problems.

There has been a great deal of consolidation in healthcare. There have been over 1,500 hospital mergers in the past 20 years, with nearly 700 since 2010.

The result is that many local areas are now dominated by one large, powerful healthcare system, such as Boston with Partners Health, Pittsburgh with University of Pittsburgh Medical Center, and the San Francisco Bay area with Sutter.

Insurance markets are also highly consolidated. The two largest insurers have 70 percent or more of the market and more than one-half of all local insurance markets.

Physician services markets have also become increasingly consolidated. Two-thirds of specialized physician markets are highly concentrated and 29 percent for primary care physicians.

There have been a very, very large number of acquisitions of physician practices by hospitals, so much so that one-third of all physicians and 44 percent of primary care physicians are now employed by hospitals.

There are a number of reasons for this consolidation, and of course they vary across transactions. These include attempts to enhance or entrench market position in order to maintain or increase rates, revenue, and profits to protect market share.

There are also what one could call Newton's Third Law of Consolidation—for every action, there is an equal and opposite reaction. If payers consolidate, then insurance companies feel they must consolidate to protect their position. Providers then feel they must consolidate and so on, and you can have a vicious cycle, not a virtuous cycle, of consolidation for strategic reasons, not for reasons to improve the quality of care or help patients.

Their responses to financial incentives unintended in payment policies, specifically site-specific payments for the same physician service, can be double or larger if a physician practice is owned by a hospital, and the

340B program makes drug discounts available to hospitals but not to independent physician practices.

There are legitimate efforts to achieve scale for lower cost, avoid unnecessary duplication, accepting risk-based payments, better coordinate care, facilitate investments in care coordination and quality.

There are also concerns about the future. There's been a great deal of upheaval in healthcare over the past few years for a variety of reasons, and sometimes entities feel that they are protecting themselves by consolidation.

Last, one should be aware that there is a global merger wave happening, and there are many mergers throughout our economy. So there are undoubtedly factors that are not specific to healthcare but that have to do with what's happening in the economy as a whole.

Extensive research evidence shows that consolidation between close competitors leads to substantial price increases for hospitals, insurers, and physicians without offsetting gains in improved quality or enhanced efficiency.

Further, recent evidence shows that mergers between hospitals not in the same geographic area can also lead to increases in price. Just as seriously if not more so, evidence shows that patient quality of care suffers from lack of competition.

Lack of competition and consolidation entrenches existing modes of organization and delivery of care and prevents the emerging of new and innovative ways of organizing care.

Policies are needed to support and promote competition in healthcare markets. This includes policies to strengthen choice and competition and ending distortions that unintentionally incentivize consolidation.

Now, there's no one policy that will achieve all of these. Rather, we need a constellation of policies that will work to mutually reinforce each other.

These include focusing and strengthening antitrust enforcement, ending policies that unintentionally incentivize consolidation, ending policies that hamper new competitors and impede competition, promoting transparency so employers, policy makers, and consumers have access to information about healthcare costs and quality.

We are facing a great challenge to our healthcare system. If left unchecked, consolidation could undermine our best efforts to control costs, improve care, and make our system more responsive and dynamic.

We need new and vigorous policies to encourage beneficial organizational change and innovation. If we fail, we will likely have an even more expensive, less responsive health system that will be exceedingly hard to change.

In my opinion, this is the number-one priority for healthcare. The time to act is now.

Thank you.

[The statement of Dr. Gaynor follows:]

EXAMINING THE IMPACT OF HEALTH CARE CONSOLIDATION, STATEMENT BEFORE THE COMMITTEE ON ENERGY AND COMMERCE OVERSIGHT AND INVESTIGATIONS SUBCOMMITTEE, U.S. HOUSE OF REPRESENTATIVES

by Martin Gaynor, E.J. Barone University Professor of Economics and Health Policy, Heinz College, Carnegie Mellon University, Washington, D.C., February 14, 2018

Summary of Statement

- The U.S. health care system is based on markets. The system will work only as well as the markets that underpin it.
- These markets do not function as well as they could, or should. Prices are high and rising, there are incomprehensible and egregious pricing practices, quality is suboptimal, and the sector is

sluggish and unresponsive, in contrast to the innovation and dynamism which characterize much of the rest of our economy.
- Lack of competition has a lot to do with these problems.
- There has been a great deal of consolidation in health care. There have been 1,519 hospital mergers in the past twenty years, with 680 since 2010. The result is that many local areas are now dominated by one large, powerful health system, e.g., Boston (Partners), Pittsburgh (UPMC), and San Francisco (Sutter).
- Insurance markets are also highly consolidated. The two largest insurers have 70 percent of the market or more in one-half of all local insurance markets.
- Physician services markets have also become increasingly more concentrated. Two-thirds of specialist physician markets are highly concentrated, and 29 percent for primary care physicians. There have been a very large number of acquisitions of physician practices by hospitals, so much so that 33 percent of all physicians, and 44 percent of primary physicians are now employed by hospitals.
- Extensive research evidence shows that consolidation between close competitors leads to substantial price increases for hospitals, insurers, and physicians, without offsetting gains in improved quality or enhanced efficiency. Further, recent evidence shows that mergers between hospitals not in the same geographic area can also lead to increases in price. Just as seriously, if not more, evidence shows that patient quality of care suffers from lack of competition.
- This is causing serious harm to patients and to the health care system as a whole.
- Policies are needed to support and promote competition in health care markets. This includes policies to strengthen choice and competition, and ending distortions that unintentionally incentivize consolidation.
- These include:
    - Focus and strengthen antitrust enforcement.

- End policies that unintentionally incentivize consolidation.
- End policies that hamper new competitors and impede competition.
- Promote transparency, so employers, policymakers, and consumers have access to information about health care costs and quality.

Statement

Chairman Harper, Ranking Member DeGette, and Members of the Subcommittee, thank you for holding a hearing on this vitally important topic and for giving me the opportunity to testify in front of you today.

1. My Background

I am an economist who has been studying the health care sector, and specifically health care markets and competition, for nearly 40 years. I am a Professor of Economics and Public Policy at the Heinz College of Public Policy at Carnegie Mellon University in Pittsburgh. I served as the Director of the Bureau of Economics at the Federal Trade Commission during 2013-2014, during which time I was involved in the many health care matters that came before the Commission. I have also served the Commonwealth of Pennsylvania as a member of the Governor's Health Advisory Board and as Co-Chair of its Working Group on Shoppable Health Care.

I am currently engaged in research that is directly relevant to the topic of this hearing. My project with colleagues Zack Cooper, Stuart Craig, and John Van Reenen exploits newly available data on nearly 90 million individuals with private, employer sponsored health insurance nationwide to examine variation in health care spending and prices for the privately insured (Cooper et al., 2015). One of our key findings is that hospitals that have fewer potential competitors nearby have substantially higher prices. For example, monopoly hospitals' prices are on average 12.5 percent higher than hospitals with 3 or more potential competitors nearby. The prices of hospitals who have one other nearby potential competitor are on average 7.6 percent higher. We also examine all hospital mergers in the United States over a five year period, and find that the average merger between two nearby hospitals (5 miles or closer) leads to a price increase of 6.2 percent. Further, our evidence shows that prices continue to rise for at least two years after the merger. Last, we find that hospitals that face fewer competitors can negotiate more favorable forms of payments, and resist those they dislike – a serious issue for payment reform.

My papers with Katherine Ho and Robert Town, "The Industrial Organization of Health Care Market," (Gaynor et al., 2015), with Robert Town, "Competition in Health Care Markets," (Gaynor and Town, 2012a), and my with Robert Town "The Impact of Hospital Consolidation: Update" (Gaynor and Town, 2012b) are also relevant to the topic of this hearing. In those papers my co-authors and I review the research evidence on health care markets and competition. We find that there is extensive evidence that competition leads to lower prices, and often improves quality, whereas consolidation between close competitors does the opposite.

My recent White Paper with Farzad Mostashari and Paul Ginsburg (Gaynor et al., 2017) is also directly relevant to the topic of this hearing. In this White Paper Mostashari, Ginsburg, and I identify factors that are impeding the effective functioning of health care markets and propose a number of actionable solutions to make health care markets work better.

2. Introduction

Health care is a very large and important industry. Health care spending is now over $3.3 trillion and accounts for approximately 18 percent of GDP – nearly one-fifth of the entire U.S. economy (Hartman et al., 2018). Hospital and physician services are a large part of the U.S. economy. In 2016, hospital care alone accounted for almost one-third of total health spending and 5.8% of GDP – roughly twice the size of automobile manufacturing, agriculture, or mining, and larger than all manufacturing sectors except food and beverage and tobacco products, which is approximately the same size. Physician services comprise 3.6% of

GDP (Hartman et al., 2018). The net cost of health insurance – current year premiums minus current year medical benefits paid – was 1.2% of GDP in 2016. The share of the economy accounted for by these sectors has risen dramatically over the last 30 years. In 1980, hospitals and physicians accounted for 3.6% and 1.7% of U.S. GDP, respectively, while the net cost of health insurance in 1980 was 0.34% (Martin et al., 2011).

Of course, health care is important not only because of its size. Health care services can save lives or dramatically affect the quality of life, thereby substantially improving well being and productivity.

As a consequence, the functioning of the health care sector is vitally important. A well functioning health care sector is an asset to the economy and improves quality of life for the citizenry. By the same token, problems in the health care sector act as a drag on the economy and impose a burden on individuals.

The U.S. health care system is based on markets. The vast majority of health care is privately provided (with some exceptions, such as public hospitals, the Veterans Administration, and the Indian Health Service) and over half of health care is privately financed (Hartman et al., 2018). As a consequence, the health care system will only work as well as the markets that underpin it. If those markets function poorly, then we will get health care that's not as good as it could be and that costs more than it should. Moreover, attempts at reform, no matter how important or clever, will not prove successful if they are built on top of dysfunctional markets.

There is widespread agreement that these markets do not work as well as they could, or should. Prices are high and rising (Rosenthal, 2017; National Academy of Social Insurance, 2015; New York State Health Foundation, 2016), they vary in seemingly incoherent ways, there are egregious pricing practices (Cooper and Scott Morton, 2016; Rosenthal, 2017), there are serious concerns about the quality of care (Institute of Medicine, 2001; Kohn et al., 1999; Kessler and McClellan, 2000), and the system is sluggish and unresponsive, lacking the innovation and dynamism that characterize much of the rest of our economy (Cutler, 2010; Chin et al., 2015; Herzlinger, 2006).

One of the reasons for this is lack of competition. The research evidence shows that hospitals and doctors who face less competition charge higher prices to private payers, without accompanying gains in efficiency or quality. Research shows the same for insurance markets. Insurers who face less competition charge higher premiums, and may pay lower prices to providers. Moreover, the evidence also shows that lack of competition can cause serious harm to the quality of care received by patients.

It's important to recognize that the burden of higher provider prices falls on individuals, not insurers or employers. Health care is not like commodity products, such as milk or gasoline. If the price of milk or gasoline go up, consumers experience directly when they purchase these products. However, even though individuals with private employer provided health insurance pay a small portion of provider fees directly out of their own pockets, they end up paying for increased prices in the end. Insurers facing higher provider prices increase their premiums to employers. Employers then pass those increased premiums on to their workers, either in the form of lower wages (or smaller wage increases) or reduced benefits (greater premium sharing or less extensive coverage, including the loss of coverage) (Gruber, 1994; Bhattacharya and Bundorf, 2005; Baicker and Chandra, 2006; Emanuel and Fuchs, 2008; Baicker and Chandra, 2006; Currie and Madrian, 2000; Anand, 2017). As mentioned previously, when consolidation leads to providers obtaining higher prices from providers the impact ultimately falls on consumers, not insurers or employers. Figure 1 illustrates this. Workers' contributions to health insurance premiums grew 242 percent from 1999 to 2016, while wages grew by only 60 percent.

The burden of private health care spending on U.S. households has been growing, so much so that it's taking up a larger and larger share of household spending and exceeding increases in pay for many workers. Figure 2 illustrates that middle class families' spending on health care has increased 25 percent since 2007, crowding out spending on other goods and services, including food, housing, and clothing. Health insurance fringe benefits for workers, chief among which is health care, increased as a share of workers' total compensation over this same period, growing from 12 to 14.5 percent, while wages stayed flat (see Monaco and Pierce, 2015, Table 1).

As documented below, there has been a tremendous amount of consolidation among health care providers. Consolidation has also been occurring among health insurers. It's important to be clear that consolidation can be either beneficial or harmful. Consolidation can bring efficiencies – it can reduce inefficient duplication of services, allow firms to combine to achieve efficient size, or facilitate investment in quality or efficiency improvements. Successful firms may also expand by acquiring others. If firms get larger by being better at giving consumers what they want or driving down costs so their goods are cheaper, that's a good thing (big does not equal bad), so long as they don't engage in actions to attempt to then limit competition. On the other hand, consolidation can reduce competition and enhance market power and thereby lead to increased prices or reduced quality.

3. Consolidation

There has been a tremendous amount of consolidation in the health care industry over the last 20 years. A recent paper by Fulton (2017) documents these trends and shows high and increasing concentration in U.S. hospital, physician, and insurance markets. Figure 5 illustrates these trends from 2010 to 2016, using the Herfindahl-Hirschman Index (HHI) measure of market concentration.[1]

3.1. Hospitals

The American Hospital Association documents 1,412 hospital mergers from 1998 to 2015, with 561 occurring from 2010 to 2015. Figure 3 illustrates the number of mergers and the number of hospitals involved in these transactions from 1998 to 2015. A trade publication documents an

---

[1] The HHI is equal to the sum of firms' market shares. It reaches a maximum of 10,000 when there is only one firm in the market. It gets smaller the more equal are firms' market shares and the more firms there are in the market.

additional 115 hospital mergers in 2017 and 102 in 2016 and 2017 (Kaufman Hall, 2018).

While some of these mergers may have little or no impact on competition, many include mergers between close competitors, especially given that hospital markets are already highly concentrated. Figure 4 shows that almost half of the hospital mergers occurring from 2010 to 2012 were between hospitals in the same area.[2] Further, as indicated below, recent evidence indicates that even mergers between hospitals in different may lead to higher priceas.

As a result of this consolidation, the majority of hospital markets are highly concentrated, and many areas of the country are dominated by one or two large hospital systems with no close competitors (Cutler and Scott Morton, 2013; Fulton, 2017).[3] This includes places like Boston (Partners), Cleveland (Cleveland Clinic and University Hospital), Pittsburgh (UPMC), and San Francisco (Sutter). Mergers that eliminate close competitors cause direct harm to competition. In addition, once a firm has obtained a dominant position it often engages in anticompetitive practices in order to maintain it.

3.2. Physicians

Capps et al. (2017) find that there has been major consolidation among physician practices. Physician practices with 11 or more doctors grew larger from 2007 to 2013, mainly through acquisitions of smaller physician practices, while practices with 10 or fewer doctors grew smaller. Muhlestein and Smith (2016) also report that the proportion of physicians in small practices dropped from 2013 to 2015, while the proportion in large practices increased. Kane (2017) reports similar trends. Fulton (2017) reports that 65 percent of MSAs were highly concentrated for specialist physicians, and 39 percent for primary care physicians. He finds a

---

[2] The areas used are Core Based Statistical Areas. For a definition see (p. A-15 in U.S. Census Bureau, 2012).
[3] Fulton (2017) reports that 90 percent of Metropolitan Statistical Areas (MSAs) were highly concentrated for hospitals. Highly concentrated means an HHI of 2,500 or greater. The U.S. antitrust enforcement agencies define an HHI of 2,500 or above as "highly concentrated" (Federal Trade Commission and Department of Justice, 1992).

particularly pronounced increase in market concentration for primary care physicians.

Moreover, there have been a very large number of acquisitions of physician practices by hospitals. In 2006, 28 percent of primary physicians were employed by hospitals. By 2016, that number had risen to 44 percent (Fulton, 2017). The American Medical Association reports that 33 percent of all physicians were employed by hospitals in 2016, and less than half own their own practice (Kane, 2017). Fulton (2017) finds that increased concentration in primary care physician markets is associated with practices being owned by hospitals.

3.3. Insurers

The insurance industry is also highly concentrated. Fulton (2017) finds that 57 percent of health insurance markets were highly concentrated in 2016. The American Medical Association reports that 69 percent were highly concentrated (American Medical Association, 2017). The market share of the top four insurers in the fully insured commercial segment was 76 percent in 2013, up from 61 percent in 2001 (see Figure 6). If one looks at the state or local level, the concentration is more pronounced. In 2014, the two largest insurers had 70 percent or more of the market in one half of all MSAs (Figure 7).

4. Evidence on the Impacts of Consolidation

There is now a considerable body of scientific research evidence on the impacts of consolidation in health care. Most of the research studies are on the hospital sector, because data have typically been more readily available for hospitals than for physicians or for insurers, but there are now a considerable number of research studies on those industries as well (see Gaynor et al., 2015; Gaynor and Town, 2012a,b; Dranove and Satterthwaite, 2000; Gaynor and Vogt, 2000; Vogt and Town, 2006, for reviews of the evidence).

4.1. Impacts on Prices

4.1.1. Hospitals

There are many studies of hospital mergers. These studies look at many different mergers in different places in different time periods, and find substantial increases in price resulting from mergers in concentrated markets (Haas-Wilson and Garmon, 2011; Tenn, 2011; Thompson, 2011; Dafny, 2009; Krishnan, 2001; Vita and Sacher, 2001; Capps and Dranove, 2004; Gowrisankaran et al., 2015; Gaynor and Vogt, 2003; Town and Vistnes, 2001; Capps et al., 2003). Price increases on the order of 20 or 30 percent are common, and can range to over 50 percent.

These results make sense. Hospitals' negotiations with insurers determine prices and whether they are in an insurer's provider network. Insurers want to build a provider network that employers (and consumers) will value. If two hospitals are viewed as good alternatives to each other by consumers (close substitutes), then the insurer can substitute one for the other with little loss to the value of their product, and therefore each hospital's bargaining leverage is limited. If one hospital declines to join the network, customers will be "almost as happy" with access to the other. If the two hospitals merge, the insurer will now lose substantial value if they offer a network without the merged entity (if there are no other hospitals viewed as good alternatives by consumers). The merger therefore generates bargaining leverage and hospitals can negotiate a price increase.

Overall, these studies consistently show that when hospital consolidation is between close competitors it raises prices, and by substantial amounts. Consolidated hospitals that are able to charge higher prices due to reduced competition are able to do so on an ongoing basis, making this a permanent rather than a transitory problem.

There is also more recent evidence that mergers between hospitals that are not near to each other can lead to price increases. Quite a few hospital mergers are between hospitals that are not in the same area (see Figure 4). Many employers have locations with employees in a number of geographic areas. These employers will most likely prefer insurance plans with provider networks that cover their employees in all of these locations. An insurance plan thus has an incentive to have a provider network that covers the multiple locations of employers. It is therefore costly for that insurer to lose a hospital system that has hospitals in multiple locations – their network would become less attractive. This means that a merger between hospitals in these locations can increase their bargaining power, and hence their prices.

There are two recent papers find evidence that such mergers lead to significant hospital price increases. Lewis and Pflum (2017) find that such mergers lead to price increases of 17 percent. Dafny et al. (2017) find that mergers between hospitals in different markets in the same state (but not in different states) lead to price increases of 10 percent.

This is an important area for further investigation, and determining appropriate policy responses.

4.1.2. Physicians

There is also substantial evidence that physician practices facing less competition have substantially higher prices. Koch and Ulrick (2017) examine the effects of a merger of six orthopedic groups in southeastern Pennsylvania and find that the merger generated large price increases – nearly 25 percent for one payer and 15 percent for another. Dunn and Shapiro (2014), Baker et al. (2014b), Austin and Baker (2015) all find that physician practices that face fewer potential competitors have substantially higher prices.

Moreover, studies that examine the impacts of hospital acquisitions of physician practices find that such acquisitions result in significantly higher prices and more spending (Capps et al., 2016; Neprash et al., 2015; Baker et al., 2014a; Robinson and Miller, 2014). For example, Capps et al. (2016) find that hospital acquisitions of physician practices led to prices increasing by an average of 14 percent and patient spending increasing by 4.9 percent.

4.1.3. Insurers

Insurance premiums also respond strongly to competition. Markets with more insurers have substantially lower premiums. Insurer premiums are driven in large part by medical expenses. Premiums cover the majority of health care expenses of enrollees, so factors that increase health care spending also increase health insurance premiums. However, the cost of private health insurance net of medical expenses also has grown rapidly in recent years (12.4 percent in 2014 and 7.6 percent in 2016), such that health insurance costs comprised 6.6 percent of total health spending in 2015, compared to 5.5 percent in 2009 (Martin et al., 2016). Further, there is substantial geographic variation in health insurance premiums. For example, premiums for an individual silver plan in the ACA marketplaces ranged from $163 to $1,119 per month (Robert Wood Johnson Foundation, HIX Compare https://hixcompare.org).

Research evidence indicates that premiums are higher in more consolidated insurance markets, leading to concerns about competition among insurers and about increasing consolidation (Dafny, 2015, 2010; Dafny et al., 2012). For example, the merger between Aetna and Prudential in 1999 was found to have led to a 7 percent increase in premiums for large employers. Similarly, the Sierra United merger in 2008 was found to have led to an almost 14 percent increase in small group premiums (Guardado et al., 2013). Moreover, researchers have found that adding one more insurer to an ACA marketplace reduces premiums by 4.5 percent (Dafny et al., 2015), and that eliminating an insurer for an employer to choose from can lead to large (16.6 percent) premium increases (Ho and Lee, 2017).

4.2. Impacts on Quality

Just as, if not more, important than impacts on prices are impacts on the quality of care. The quality of health care can have profound impacts on patients' lives, including their probability of survival.

4.2.1. Hospitals

A number of studies have found that patient health outcomes are substantially worse at hospitals in more concentrated markets, where those hospitals face less potential competition.

Studies of markets with administered prices (e.g., Medicare) find that less competition leads to worse quality. One of the most striking results is from Kessler and McClellan (2000), who find that risk-adjusted one year mortality for Medicare heart attack (acute myocardial infarction, or AMI) patients is significantly higher in more concentrated markets.[4] In particular, patients in the most concentrated markets had mortality probabilities 1.46 points higher than those in the least concentrated markets (this constitutes a 4.4% difference) as of 1991. This is an extremely large difference – it amounts to over 2,000 fewer (statistical) deaths in the least concentrated vs. most concentrated markets.

There are similar results from studies of the English National Health Service (NHS). The NHS adopted a set of reforms in 2006 that were intended to increase patient choice and hospital competition, and introduced administered prices for hospitals based on patient diagnoses (analogous to the Medicare Prospective Payment System). Two recent studies examine the impacts of this reform (Cooper et al., 2011; Gaynor et al., 2013) and find that, following the reform, risk-adjusted mortality from heart attacks fell more at hospitals in less concentrated markets than at hospitals in more concentrated markets. Gaynor et al. (2013) also look at mortality from all causes and find that patients fared worse at hospitals in more consolidated markets.

Studies of markets where prices are market determined (e.g., markets for those with private health insurance) find that consolidation can lead to lower quality, although some studies go the other way. Romano and Balan (2011) find that the merger of Evanston Northwestern and Highland Park hospitals had no effect on some quality indicators, while it harmed others. Capps (2005) finds that hospital mergers in New York state had no impacts on many quality indicators, but led to increases in mortality for patients suffering from heart attacks and from failure. Cutler et al. (2010) find that the removal of barriers to entry led to increased market shares for low mortality rate CABG surgeons in Pennsylvania.

---

[4] Concentrated markets have fewer competitors or are dominated by a small number of competitors, e.g., one large hospital.

4.2.2. Physicians

There is also evidence that the quality of care delivered by physicians suffers when physician practices face less competition. Koch et al. (2018) find that an increase in consolidation among cardiology practices leads to increases in negative health outcomes for their patients. They find that moving from a zip code at the 25th percentile of the cardiology market concentration to one at the 75th percentile is associated with 5 to 7 percent increases in risk-adjusted mortality. Eisenberg (2011) finds that cardiologists who face less competition have patients with higher mortality rates. McWilliams et al. (2013) find that larger hospital owned physician practices have higher readmission rates and perform no better than smaller practices on process based measures of quality. Roberts et al. (2017) find that quality of care at high priced physicians practices is no better than at low priced physician practices. Further, the testimony of Dr. Kenneth Kizer in a recent physician practice merger case documents that clinical integration is achieved with many different forms of organization, i.e., that consolidation isn't necessary to achieve the benefits of clinical integration.[5]

4.3. Impacts on Costs, Coordination, Quality

It is plausible that consolidation between hospital, physician practices or insurers, in a number of combinations, could reduce costs, increase care coordination, or enhance efficiency. There may be gains from operating at a larger scale, eliminating wasteful duplication, improved communications, enhanced incentives for mutually beneficial investments, etc. However, it is important to realize that consolidation is not integration. Acquiring another firm changes ownership, but in and of itself does nothing to achieve integration. Integration, if it happens, is a long process that occurs after acquisition.

While the intuition, and the rhetoric, surrounding consolidation, has been positive, the reality is less encouraging. The evidence on the effects of consolidation is mixed, but it's safe to say that it does not show overall gains from consolidation. Merged hospitals, insurers, physician practices,

---

[5] https://www.ftc.gov/system/files/documents/cases/131021stlukedemokizer.pdf.

or integrated systems are not systematically less costly, higher quality, or more effective than independent firms (see Burns and Muller, 2008; Burns et al., 2015; Goldsmith et al., 2015; Burns et al., 2013; McWilliams et al., 2013; Tsai and Jha, 2014). For example, Burns et al. (2015) find no evidence that hospital systems are lower cost, Goldsmith et al. (2015) find no evidence that integrated delivery systems perform better than independents, Koch et al. (2018) find higher Medicare expenditures for cardiology practices in consolidated markets, and McWilliams et al. (2013) find higher Medicare expenditures for large hospital-based practices. Since consolidation in health care has been occurring for a long time, it seems unlikely that the promised gains from consolidation will now materialize if they haven't yet.

5. Policies to Make Health Care Markets Work

As I have discussed, consolidation in health care has not delivered on lower costs, improved coordination of care, or enhanced quality. What has happened is that consolidation between hospitals, physician practices, and insurers who are close competitors has reduced competition, leading to higher prices and harming quality. Even worse, reduced competition tends to preserve the status quo in health care by protecting existing firms and making it more difficult for new firms to enter markets and succeed. This leads to excessive rigidity and resistance to change, as opposed to the innovation and dynamism that we need.

Farzad Mostashari, Paul Ginsburg and I have proposed a set of policies to enhance competition in health care (Gaynor et al., 2017). Rather than recapping what has already been written, let me briefly summarize some key points, and add a few new thoughts.

- One key set of actions is to end policies that unintentionally provide incentives for consolidation. It has been well documented that certain Medicare payment policies have the unintended effect of doing this. Putting an end to policies that artificially encourage consolidation will help by reducing consolidation, and thereby consolidation that harms competition along with it.

- Another set of things that can be done to reduce unintended incentives to consolidate is to reduce administrative burdens that generate more costs than benefits. One example of these is quality reporting. Multiple entities: Medicare, Medicaid, multiple private insurers require provider reporting of a large set of quality measures. Coordination among payers could reduce administrative burden and thereby reduce incentives to consolidate.
- Some states have regulations that unintentionally make it difficult for new firms to enter or artificially alter the negotiating positions of providers and payers. These include certificate of need laws, any willing provider laws, scope of practice laws, and licensing board decisions. States can consider altering or eliminating these laws, or clarifying that if retained they should be limited in focus to their stated purpose.
- This also applies to state certificate of public advantage legislation. These laws, when passed, shield merging parties from federal antitrust scrutiny and impose state supervision. If certificates of public advantage continue to be issued, omitting provisions that exempt merging parties from antitrust scrutiny will help to preserve competition.
- Federal and state agencies can pursue and prevent practices that are intended to limit competition. For example, anti-tiering, anti-steering, and gag clauses prevent insurers from providing information to enrollees about more or less expensive providers, or from providing incentives to enrollees to go to less expensive providers. The federal antitrust enforcement agencies and state attorneys general can pursue these and other anticompetitive practices. In addition, state insurance commissioners can review contracts between insurers and providers and scrutinize them for clauses that harm competition and consumers.
- Transparency about health care costs and quality can be enhanced. At present there are no national, publicly available data on total U.S. health care costs and utilization, let alone on prices for specific services or providers. Data and information are now as

vital a part of our national infrastructure as are our bridges and roads. It's time to invest in a national health care data warehouse that brings together private and public data to inform employers, policymakers, and consumers.

- Antitrust enforcement in health care by federal and state governments, both horizontal and vertical, needs to be continued and enhanced. Of course if we expect the antitrust enforcement agencies to do more in health care without reducing their efforts in the rest of the economy, then they will need more resources. There are also discussions about legislation to strengthen antitrust, specifically that horizontal mergers that meet certain criteria about market structure would be presumptively illegal, and the burden would shift to defendants to establish that they are not. If this comes to pass it would strengthen the antitrust enforcment agencies' positions in dealing with health care mergers they judge to be harmful, as well as mergers in general.

Bibliography

American Medical Association (2017). Competition in health insurance: A comprehensive study of U.S. markets, 2017 update. Technical report, American Medical Association, Chicago, IL.

Anand, P. (2017). Health insurance costs and employee compensation: Evidence from the national compensation survey. *Health Economics*, 26(12):1601–1616. hec.3452.

Austin, D. and Baker, L. (2015). Less physician practice competition is associated with higher prices paid for common procedures. *Health Affairs*, 34(10):1753–1760.

Baicker, K. and Chandra, A. (2006). The labor market effects of rising health insurance premiums. *Journal of Labor Economics*, 24(3):609–634.

Baker, L., Bundorf, M., and Kessler, D. (2014a). Vertical integration: Hospital ownership of physician practices is associated with higher prices and spending. *Health Affairs*, 33(5):756–763.

Baker, L., Bundorf, M., Royalty, A., and Levin, Z. (2014b). Physician practice competition and prices paid by private insurers for office visits. *JAMA*, 312(16):1653–1662.

Bhattacharya, J. and Bundorf, M. K. (2005). The incidence of the healthcare costs of obesity. National Bureau of Economic Research Working Paper No. 11303.

Burns, L., McCullough, J., Wholey, D., Kruse, G., Kralovec, P., and Muller, R. (2015). Is the system really the solution? Operating costs in hospital systems. *Medical Care Research and Review*, 72(3):247–272.

Burns, L. and Muller, R. (2008). Hospital-physician collaboration: Landscape of economic integration and impact on clinical integration. *Milbank Quarterly*, 86(3):375–434.

Burns, L. R., Goldsmith, J., and Sen, A. (2013). Horizontal and vertical integration of physicians: A tale of two tails. *Annual Review of Health Care Management: Revisiting the Evolution of Health Systems Organization Advances in Health Care Management*, 15:39–117.

Capps, C. (2005). The quality effects of hospital mergers. unpublished manuscript, Bates White LLC.

Capps, C. and Dranove, D. (2004). Hospital consolidation and negotiated PPO prices. *Health Affairs*, 23(2):175–181.

Capps, C., Dranove, D., and Ody, C. (2016). The effect of hospital acquisitions of physician practices on prices and spending. unpublished manuscript, Northwestern University.

Capps, C., Dranove, D., and Ody, C. (2017). Physician practice consolidation driven by small acquisitions, so antitrust agencies have few tools to intervene. *Health Affairs*, 36(9):1556–1563.

Capps, C., Dranove, D., and Satterthwaite, M. (2003). Competition and market power in option demand markets. *RAND Journal of Economics*, 34(4):737–63.

Chin, W., Hamermesh, R., Huckman, R., McNeil, B., and Newhouse, J. (2015). 5 imperatives addressing health care's innovation challenge.

Technical report, Forum on Healthcare Innovation. Harvard University, Boston, MA.

Cooper, Z., Craig, S., Gaynor, M., and Van Reenen, J. (2015). The price ain't right? Hospital prices and health spending on the privately insured. Working Paper 21815, National Bureau of Economic Research, Cambridge, MA.

Cooper, Z., Gibbons, S., Jones, S., and McGuire, A. (2011). Does hospital competition save lives? evidence from the English NHS patient choice reforms. *The Economic Journal*, 121(554):F228–F260.

Cooper, Z. and Scott Morton, F. (2016). Out-of-network emergency-physician bills – An unwelcome surprise. *New England Journal of Medicine*, 375(20):1915–1918.

Currie, J. and Madrian, B. (2000). Health, health insurance, and the labor market. In Ashenfelter, O. and Card, D., editors, *Handbook of Labor Economics*, pages 3309–3416. Elsevier Science, Amsterdam.

Cutler, D. (2010). Where are the health care entrepreneurs? The failure of organizational innovation in health care. *Innovation Policy and the Economy*, 11(1):1 – 28. http://www.journals.uchicago.edu/doi/10.1 086/655816.

Cutler, D. M., Huckman, R. S., and Kolstad, J. T. (2010). Input constraints and the efficiency of entry: Lessons from cardiac surgery. *American Economic Journal: Economic Policy*, 2(1):51–76.

Cutler, D. M. and Scott Morton, F. (2013). Hospitals, market share, and consolidation. *JAMA*, 310(18):1964–1970. http://jamanetwork.com/journals/jama/article-abstract/1769891.

Dafny, L. (2009). Estimation and identification of merger effects: An application to hospital mergers. *Journal of Law and Economics*, 52(3):pp. 523–550.

Dafny, L. (2010). Are health insurance markets competitive? *American Economic Review*, 100:1399–1431.

Dafny, L. (2015). Evaluating the impact of health insurance industry consolidation: Learning from experience. Issue brief, The Commonwealth Fund, New York, NY.

Dafny, L., Duggan, M., and Ramanarayanan, S. (2012). Paying a premium on your premium? Consolidation in the U.S. health insurance industry. *American Economic Review*, 102(2):1161–1185.

Dafny, L., Gruber, J., and Ody, C. (2015). More insurers lower premiums: Evidence from initial pricing in the health insurance marketplaces. *American Journal of Health Economics*, 1(1):53–81.

Dafny, L., Ho, K., and Lee, R. (2017). The price effects of cross-market mergers: Theory and evidence from the hospital industry. unpublished manuscript, http://www.columbia.edu/kh2214/papers/DafnyHoLee062717.pdf.

Dranove, D. D. and Satterthwaite, M. A. (2000). The industrial organization of health care markets. In Culyer, A. and Newhouse, J., editors, *Handbook of Health Economics*, chapter 20, pages 1094–1139. Elsevier Science, North-Holland, New York and Oxford.

Dunn, A. and Shapiro, A. (2014). Do physicians possess market power? *Journal of Law and Economics*, 57(1):159–193.

Eisenberg, M. (2011). Reimbursement rates and physician participation in Medicare. unpublished manuscript, Carnegie Mellon University.

Emanuel, E. and Fuchs, V. R. (2008). Who really pays for health care? The myth of "shared responsibility." *Journal of the American Medical Association*, 299(9):1057–1059.

Federal Trade Commission and Department of Justice (1992). Horizontal merger guidelines. Issued April 2, 1992, Revised September, 2010.

Fulton, B. D. (2017). Health care market concentration trends in the United States: Evidence and policy responses. *Health Affairs*, 36(9):1530–1538.

Gaynor, M., Ho, K., and Town, R. J. (2015). The industrial organization of health care markets. *Journal of Economic Literature*, 53(2):235–284.

Gaynor, M., Moreno-Serra, R., and Propper, C. (2013). Death by market power: Reform, competition and patient outcomes in the National Health Service. *American Economic Journal: Economic Policy*, 5(4):134–166.

Gaynor, M., Mostashari, F., and Ginsburg, P. B. (2017). Making health care markets work: Competition policy for health care. White paper,

Heinz College, Carnegie Mellon; Brookings Institution; Robert Wood Johnson Foundation. available at http://www.brookings.edu.

Gaynor, M. and Town, R. J. (2012a). Competition in health care markets. In McGuire, T. G., Pauly, M. V., and Pita Barros, P., editors, *Handbook of Health Economics*, volume 2, chapter 9. Elsevier North-Holland, Amsterdam and London.

Gaynor, M. and Town, R. J. (2012b). The impact of hospital consolidation: Update. The Synthesis Project, Policy Brief No. 9, The Robert Wood Johnson Foundation, Princeton, NJ.

Gaynor, M. and Vogt, W. (2003). Competition among hospitals. *RAND Journal of Economics*, 34:764–785.

Gaynor, M. and Vogt, W. B. (2000). Antitrust and competition in health care markets. In Culyer, A. and Newhouse, J., editors, *Handbook of Health Economics*, chapter 27, pages 1405–1487. Elsevier Science, North-Holland, New York and Oxford.

Goldsmith, J., Burns, L. R., Sen, A., and Goldsmith, T. (2015). Integrated delivery networks: In search of benefits and market effects. Report, National Academy of Social Insurance, Washington, DC.

Gowrisankaran, G., Nevo, A., and Town, R. J. (2015). Mergers when prices are negotiated: Evidence from the hospital industry. *American Economic Review*, 105(1):172?–203.

Gruber, J. (1994). The incidence of mandated maternity benefits. *American Economic Review*, 84:622–641.

Guardado, J., Emmons, D., and Kane, C. (2013). The price effects of a large merger of health insurers: A case study of UnitedHealth-Sierra. *Health Management, Policy and Innovation*.

Haas-Wilson, D. and Garmon, C. (2011). Hospital mergers and competitive effects: Two retrospective analyses. *International Journal of the Economics of Business*, 18(1):17–32.

Hartman, M., Martin, A. B., Espinosa, N., Catlin, A., and The National Health Expenditure Accounts Team (2018). National health care spending in 2016: Spending and enrollment growth slow after initial coverage expansions. *Health Affairs*, 37(1):150–160.

Herzlinger, R. (2006). Why innovation in health care is so hard. *Harvard Business Review.* https://hbr.org/2006/05/why-innovation-in-health-care-is-so-hard.

Ho, K. and Lee, R. S. (2017). Insurer competition in health care markets. *Econometrica*, 85(2):379–417.

Institute of Medicine (2001). *Crossing the Quality Chasm: A New Health System for the Twenty-First Century.* National Academy Press, Washington, D.C.

Kane, C. K. (2017). Updated data on physician practice arrangements: Physician ownership drops below 50 percent. Policy research perspectives., American Medical Association, Chicago, IL.

Kaufman Hall (2018). 2017 in review: The year M&A shook the healthcare landscape. Skokie, IL: Kaufman Hall and Associates, LLC, https://www.kaufmanhall.com/resources/2017-review-year-ma-shook-healthcare-landscape.

Kessler, D. and McClellan, M. (2000). Is hospital competition socially wasteful? *Quarterly Journal of Economics*, 115(2):577–615.

Koch, T. and Ulrick, S. (2017). Price effects of a merger: Evidence from a physicians' market. Working Paper 333, Bureau of Economics, Federal Trade Commission, Washington, DC.

Koch, T., Wendling, B., and Wilson, N. E. (2018). Physician market structure, patient outcomes, and spending: An examination of Medicare beneficiaries. *Health Services Research.* forthcoming.

Kohn, L., Corrigan, J., and Donaldson, M., editors (1999). *To Err is Human: Building a Safer Health System.* National Academy Press, Washington, DC.

Krishnan, R. (2001). Market restructuring and pricing in the hospital industry. *Journal of Health Economics*, 20:213–237.

Lewis, M. and Pflum, K. (2017). Hospital systems and bargaining power: Evidence from out-of-market acquisitions. *RAND Journal of Economics*, 48(3):579?–610.

Martin, A., Hartman, M., Washington, B., Catlin, A., and the National Health Expenditures Team (2016). National health spending: Faster growth in 2015 as coverage expands and utilization increases. *Health Affairs.*

Martin, A., Lassman, D., Whittle, L., and Catlin, A. (2011). Recession contributes to slowest annual rate of increase in health spending in five decades. *Health Affairs,* 30:111–122.

McWilliams, J. M., Chernew, M., Zaslavsky, A., Hamed, P., and Landon, B. (2013). Delivery system integration and health care spending and quality for Medicare beneficiaries. *JAMA Internal Medicine,* 173(15):1447–1456.

Monaco, K. and Pierce, B. (2015). Compensation inequality: evidence from the national compensation survey. Monthly labor review, US Bureau of Labor Statistics, Washington, DC. https://www.bls.gov/opub/mlr/2015/article/compensation-inequality-evidence-from-the-national-compensation-survey.htm.

Muhlestein, D. B. and Smith, N. J. (2016). Physician consolidation: Rapid movement from small to large group practices, 2013?15. *Health Affairs,* 35(9).

National Academy of Social Insurance (2015). Addressing pricing power in health care markets: Principles and policy options to strengthen and shape markets. Report, National Academy of Social Insurance, Washington, DC. https://www.nasi.org/research/2015/addressing-pricing-power-health-care-markets-principles-poli.

Neprash, H., Chernew, M., Hicks, A., Gibson, T., and McWilliams, J. (2015). Association of financial integration between physicians and hospitals with commercial health care prices. *JAMA Internal Medicine,* 175(12):1932–1939.

New York State Health Foundation (2016). Why are hospital prices different? An examination of New York hospital reimbursement. Report, New York State Health Foundation, New York, NY. http://nyshealthfoundation.org/resources-and-reports/resource/an-examination-of-new-york-hospital-reimbursement.

Roberts, E., Mehotra, A., and McWilliams, J. M. (2017). High-price and low-price physician practices do not differ significantly on care quality or efficiency. *Health Affairs,* 36(5):855–864.

Robinson, J. and Miller, K. (2014). Total expenditures per patient in hospital-owned and physician organizations in California. *JAMA*, 312(6):1663–1669.

Romano, P. and Balan, D. (2011). A retrospective analysis of the clinical quality effects of the acquisition of Highland Park hospital by Evanston Northwestern healthcare. *International Journal of the Economics of Business*, 18(1):45–64.

Rosenthal, E. (2017). *An American Sickness: How Healthcare became Big Business and How You Can Take it Back*. Penguin Random House, New York.

Tenn, S. (2011). The price effects of hospital mergers: A case study of the Sutter-Summit transaction. *International Journal of the Economics of Business*, 18(1):65–82.

Thompson, E. (2011). The effect of hospital mergers on inpatient prices: A case study of the New Hanover-Cape Fear transaction. *International Journal of the Economics of Business*, 18(1):91–101.

Town, R. and Vistnes, G. (2001). Hospital competition in HMO networks. *Journal of Health Economics*, 20(5):733–752.

Tsai, T. and Jha, A. (2014). Hospital consolidation, competition, and quality: Is bigger necessarily better? *JAMA*, 312(1):29 – 30. 10.1001/jama.2014.4692.

U.S. Census Bureau (2012). 2010 Census summary file 1: Technical documentation. Technical report, U.S. Census Bureau, Department of Commerce, Washington, DC. https://www.census.gov/prod/cen2010/doc/sf1.pdf#page=619.

Vita, M. and Sacher, S. (2001). The competitive effects of not-for-profit hospital mergers: A case study. *Journal of Industrial Economics*, 49(1):63–84.

Vogt, W. and Town, R. (2006). How has hospital consolidation affected the price and quality of hospital care? *Robert Wood Johnson Foundation*, pages 1–27. Policy Brief No. 9.

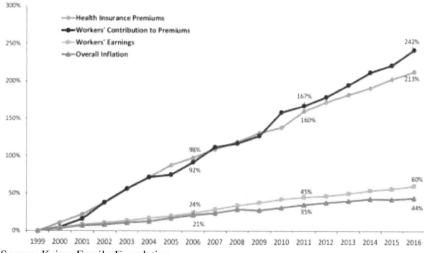

Source: Kaiser Family Foundation.

Figure 1. Growth in Health Insurance Premiums, Workers' Contributions to Premiums, Wages, and Inflation.

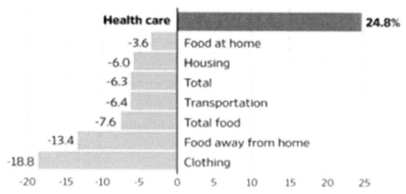

Figure 2. Change in Household Spending on Health Care and Other Basics.

Examining the Impact of Healthcare Consolidation ... 51

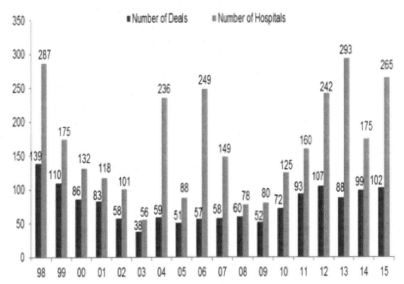

Source: American Hospital Association.

Figure 3. Number of Hospital Mergers, 1998-2015.

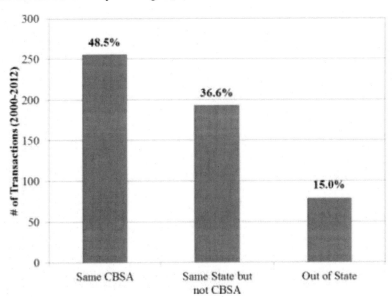

Source: Dafny et al., 2017.

Figure 4. Percent of Mergers between Hospitals in Same Area, 2010-2012.

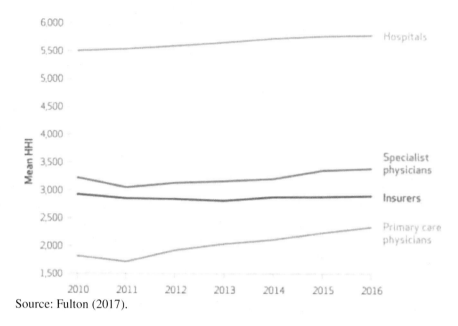

Source: Fulton (2017).

Figure 5. Market Concentration (HHI) for hospitals, physicians, and insurers, 2010-2016.

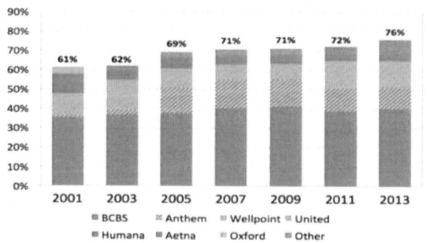

Source: Courtesy Prof. Leemore Dafny.

Figure 6. Market Share of Top 4 Insurers, Fully-Insured Commercial.

Examining the Impact of Healthcare Consolidation ... 53

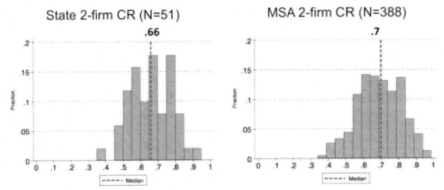

Source: Courtesy Prof. Leemore Dafny.

Figure 7. Market Share of Top 2 Insurers, Self and Full Insurance, State and MSA.

Mr. HARPER. Thank you, Dr. Gaynor.

The Chair will now recognize Dr. Dafny for 5 minutes for the purposes of an opening statement.

Thank you.

STATEMENT OF LEEMORE S. DAFNY

Dr. Dafny. Chairman Harper, Ranking Member DeGette, Representative Burgess—thank you for the kind remarks regarding my father, your professor at the University of Texas Medical School, Dr. Nachum Dafny—and all members of the subcommittee and committee.

I thank you for the opportunity to testify before you today on the subject of healthcare industry consolidation. My name is Leemore Dafny, and I am an academic health economist with longstanding research interests in competition and consolidation across a range of healthcare sectors.

I am currently the Bruce Rauner professor of business administration at the Harvard Business School and the John F. Kennedy School of Government.

Previously, I was the deputy director for healthcare and antitrust at the Bureau of Economics at the Federal Trade Commission. I serve on a panel of health advisors to the Congressional Budget Office and as a board member of not-for-profit research organizations including the American Society of Health Economists and the Healthcare Cost Institute.

As you're aware, we have seen consolidation within and across a vast array of healthcare sectors, including hospitals, health insurers, and pharmaceutical companies.

There is a substantial academic literature that finds horizontal mergers of competing healthcare providers tend to raise prices and very limited evidence to suggest there are offsetting benefits to patients in the form of improved quality.

Economists, myself included, also find that less competition among health insurers tends to raise premiums. We have less extensive evidence on combinations across different sectors.

But the evidence we have to date also finds systematic price and spending increases, in particular, after hospital systems acquire additional hospitals in the same State and after hospitals acquire physician practices.

In a nutshell, research to date suggests that consolidation in the healthcare industry on average has not yielded benefits for consumers.

Yet, I expect we'll continue to see consolidation. What drives consolidation is the expectation of a reward for the merging parties and their stakeholders. Those rewards are not likely to fall dramatically without some action.

I see four primary rewards for consolidation.

First, merging parties often improve their bargaining position, and that enhanced bargaining position can enable them to raise price and to spend the extra on either margin or mission, if they're so inclined.

Second, merging parties often believe that scale economies will produce cost savings—again, fueling margin or mission.

Third, there are reimbursement rules and programs implemented by the Centers for Medicare and Medicaid Services, CMS, that rewards certain kinds of consolidation.

And fourth, many merging parties believe common ownership will produce integrated care, which will enable them to realize synergies across the many products and services that patients require.

As I note in my written testimony, there isn't much evidence to support the beliefs regarding scale economies or integrated care, although every potential transaction needs to be evaluated on its own merits.

Merging for a better bargaining position or to game loopholes created by CMS is not value creating and often reduces value.

Achieving more competitive markets may in fact involve consolidation but only of the value-creating variety. There are steps Congress can take to promote more competitive markets.

I believe it's a worthwhile investment to create public databases containing information about the ownership and financial links among different healthcare providers and net commercial prices for their services.

This database could form the basis for regularly scheduled reports and public hearings on industry consolidation and its effects.

My counterparts with expertise on the pharmaceutical industry can advise on a similar transparency effort with respect to prescription drugs.

Second, additional funds could be appropriated to the Federal enforcement agencies for enforcement-focused research.

Third, CMS could develop alternatives to its current policies, potentially reducing the benefits for consolidation that has already been consummated.

Fourth, and most aggressive, Congress could provide financial incentives or impose regulatory requirements for employers to utilize or develop so-called private exchanges where employees can shop for their preferred health plans and make choices that reflect their own preferences.

If consumers won't pay for a higher priced product that doesn't offer greater value to warrant a price premium, the incentive to merge so as to raise price will be diminished.

Healthcare is poised to capture 1 in 5 dollars in the U.S. economy by 2020. The usual checks in place to impede anticompetitive consolidation are muted in most healthcare sectors.

To borrow from the medical vernacular, watchful waiting is not, in my opinion, the wisest approach to pursue. Sometimes a surgical intervention is necessary.

[The statement of Dr. Dafny follows:]

TESTIMONY OF LEEMORE S. DAFNY, PH.D., BRUCE V. RAUNER PROFESSOR OF BUSINESS ADMINISTRATION HARVARD BUSINESS SCHOOL, HARVARD JOHN F. KENNEDY SCHOOL OF GOVERNMENT, BEFORE THE HOUSE COMMITTEE ON ENERGY AND COMMERCE SUBCOMMITTEE ON OVERSIGHT AND INVESTIGATIONS ON "HEALTH CARE INDUSTRY CONSOLIDATION: WHAT IS HAPPENING, WHY IT MATTERS, AND WHAT PUBLIC AGENCIES MIGHT WANT TO DO ABOUT IT," FEBRUARY 14, 2018

Introduction

Chairman Harper, Ranking Member Degette, and Members of the Subcommittee, I thank you for the opportunity to testify before you today on the subject of health care industry consolidation. My name is Leemore Dafny, and I am an academic health economist with longstanding research interests in competition and consolidation across a range of healthcare sectors. I am currently the Bruce V. Rauner Professor of Business Administration at the Harvard Business School and the JFK School of Government. Previously, I held faculty positions at the Kellogg School of Management at Northwestern University, and I was the Deputy Director for Healthcare and Antitrust in the Bureau of Economics at the Federal Trade Commission. I serve on the Panel of Health Advisers to the Congressional Budget Office, and as a board member of not-for-profit research organizations including the American Society of Health Economists and the Health Care Cost Institute.

As you are aware, we have seen – and I believe we will continue to see – consolidation within and across a vast array of healthcare sectors, including hospitals, physician practices, health insurers, pharmaceutical companies, and outpatient facilities. There is a substantial academic literature that finds horizontal mergers of competing health care providers tends to raise prices, and very limited evidence to suggest there are offsetting benefits to patients in the form of improved quality. Economists, myself included, also find that less competition among health insurers tends to raise premiums. We have less extensive evidence on non-horizontal mergers in healthcare, that is mergers across providers or firms in different geographies or service categories, but the evidence we have to date also finds systematic price and spending increases, in particular after hospital systems acquire additional hospitals in the same state, and after hospitals acquire physician practices. In a nutshell, research to date suggests that consolidation in the health care industry, on average, has not yielded benefits to consumers. Yet I expect we'll continue to see more consolidation.

What drives consolidation is the expectation of a reward for the merging parties and their stakeholders. Those rewards are not likely to fall dramatically without some action. I see four primary rewards for consolidation. First, merging parties often improve their bargaining position – be it hospitals negotiating with insurers or pharmaceutical benefit managers (PBMs) negotiating with pharmaceutical companies – and that enhanced bargaining position can enable the merging parties to raise prices and to spend the extra funds on either margin or mission (if they are so inclined). Second, merging parties often believe that scale economies will produce cost savings, again fueling margin or mission. Third, there are reimbursement rules and programs implemented by the Centers for Medicare and Medicaid Services (CMS) that reward certain kinds of consolidation. Fourth, many merging parties believe common ownership will produce "integrated care," which will enable them to realize synergies across the many products and services that patients require.

As I note in my written testimony, there isn't much evidence to support the beliefs regarding scale economies or integrated care, although of course every potential transaction needs to be evaluated on its own merits.

Merging for a better bargaining position, or to game loopholes created by CMS, is not value-creating and often reduces value.

There are a steps Congress can take to promote competition in healthcare markets, which may in fact involve consolidation, but only of the "value-creating" variety. First, given the large public interest in the healthcare sector, I believe it is a worthwhile investment to create public databases containing information about the ownership and financial links among different health care providers, and net commercial prices for their services. This database could form the basis for regularly scheduled reports and public hearings on industry consolidation and its effects. My counterparts with expertise on the pharmaceutical industry can advise on a similar transparency effort with respect to prescription drugs. Second, additional funds could be appropriated to the federal enforcement agencies and earmarked for enforcement-focused research in this sector. Third, CMS could develop alternatives to its current policies, potentially reducing the benefits for consolidation that has already been consummated. Fourth, and most aggressive, Congress could provide financial incentives, or impose regulatory requirements, for employers to utilize or develop so-called "private exchanges" where employees can shop for their preferred healthplans and make choices that reflect their own preferences. Data from the public exchanges suggest consumers are more price-sensitive, and more willing to select narrow-network plans, than are employers. These preferences exert pressure on providers and healthplans to develop lower-cost health care solutions, and can therefore reduce the incentive for anticompetitive upstream mergers or practices. If consumers won't pay for a higher-priced product that doesn't offer greater value to warrant the price increase, the incentive to merge so as to raise price will be diminished.

Health care consolidation is widespread and likely to continue. The usual checks in place to impede anticompetitive consolidation are muted in most healthcare sectors. Downstream consumers are often price inelastic, partly due to the presence and design of health insurance plans and to the circumstances under which they seek and make decisions about medical care. Barriers to entry are often high and sometimes created or supported by government institutions, such as state certificate of need laws. And antitrust enforcers face legal hurdles in challenging incremental acquisitions that collectively increase the market power of acquirers, or in unwinding transactions after they have been consummated. In short, we cannot rely on the market and on antitrust enforcement to "correct" consolidation that does not deliver benefits to consumers. Healthcare is poised to capture 1 in 5 dollars of the U.S. economy by 2020. To borrow from the medical vernacular, "watchful waiting" is not – in my opinion – the wisest approach to pursue. Sometimes a surgical intervention, coupled with close monitoring and adjustments as the disease progresses, is necessary.

I. Preface: Defining Consolidation and the Scope of the Healthcare Sector

In the testimony that follows, I use the term "consolidation" to describe combinations of previously independent entities, i.e., mergers and acquisitions (M&A). One could use "consolidation" to refer to increases in the "concentration" of an industry, e.g., as measured by the sum of squared market shares (knows as the Herfindahl-Hirschman, or HHI). There are both structural and non-structural sources of consolidation. Structural changes arise from a change in the number and market share of participants (i.e., from a change in industry *structure*). Non-structural changes arise from growing (or shrinking) market shares of industry participants, holding ownership and the number of participants constant. Non-structural increases in concentration may occur, for example, if an incumbent introduces a superior product or service and customers flock to that firm and abandon others. In the interest of simplicity, I will use the term "consolidation" to refer to structurally-induced changes in concentration – specifically those generated by M&A.

The health care sector consists of a large set of industries, subdivided into the following categories in the National Health Expenditures Data: Hospital Care, Professional Services, Other Health, Residential, and Personal Care; Home Health Care; Nursing Care Facilities/Continuing

Care Retirement Communities; Retail Outlet Sales of Medical Products (prescription drugs, durable medical equipment, other non-durable medical products); Government Administration; Net Cost of Health Insurance; Government Public Health Activities; and Investment in Research and Structures/Equipment. In the testimony that follows, I focus on three of these sectors in particular: Hospital Care (32.4 percent of 2016 expenditures); Professional Services (26.4 percent); and Health Insurance (6.6 percent).[6]

II. The Facts: Where Consolidation Has Occurred, and What We Know About Its Effects

Below, I summarize the data and academic research on consolidation among healthcare providers and insurers. I subdivide my discussion into two categories: *horizontal* and *non-horizontal* consolidation. Figure 1, which depicts a simplified chain of production for one particular output of the health care sector orthopedic surgeries - provides the intuition for this division.

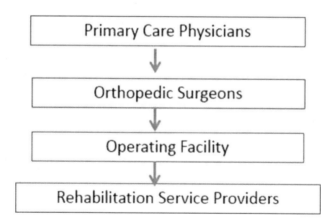

Figure 1. Vertical Chain of Production for Orthopedic Surgery.

---

[6] Centers for Medicare and Medicaid Services. NHE Fact Sheet. Retrieved from https://www.cms.gov/research-statistics-data-and-systems/statistics-trends-and-reports/nationalhealthexpenddata/nhe-fact-sheet.html.

Combinations of market participants within the same "level" of the chain are typically labeled "horizontal"; combinations up and down the chain of production are "vertical." Many healthcare markets also have a geographic element, and traditionally, the "horizontal" label is attached only to combinations in the same relevant market, e.g., a merger of two orthopedic physician practices located in the same neighborhood. Of course, combinations may have both horizontal and vertical elements (e.g., if a hospital acquires multiple physician practices and all parties are in the same geographic area), or they may fall outside these characterizations entirely (e.g., conglomerates). Given that the preponderance of data and research on consolidation has emphasized horizontal consolidation, I begin with this category, and then move to facts on non-horizontal consolidation.

II.A. Horizontal Consolidation

II.A.1. Hospitals

Most data and research on health care consolidation focuses on the hospital industry, as it is sizeable (over 5 percent of GDP, when both outpatient and inpatient services are included) and – relative to other sectors researchers have good access to data thanks to annual surveys conducted by the American Hospital Association (AHA) and to mandatory reporting through the Health Care Provider Cost Reporting Information System (HCRIS), maintained by the Centers for Medicare and Medicaid Services.

According to the AHA, the total number of hospital mergers and acquisitions (M&A) announced over the period 1998-2015 was 1,412, for an annual average of 78 transactions.[7] The pace of activity has followed a shallow U trend, with rapid activity in the late 1990s-2001, a nadir of 38 deals in 2003, and a resurgence of activity following the passage of the Affordable Care Act. In 2015, 102 deals involving 265 hospitals were

---

[7] American Hospital Association. 2016 Chart Book. Retrieved from https://www.aha.org/dataset/2018-01-17-2016-chartbook.

announced.[8] According to one recent analysis of AHA data, 90 percent of Metropolitan Statistical Areas would be characterized as "highly concentrated" per the *Horizontal Merger Guidelines* jointly issued by the DOJ and FTC (i.e., HHI above 2,500).[9]

There is a substantial body of academic research on the effects of horizontal mergers of general acute care hospitals in the U.S., and on the effects of hospital market competition in the U.S. and abroad (particularly the U.K.).[10] This research finds that mergers of competing hospitals leads to higher prices (for commercially-insured patients). There is limited evidence of quality improvements associated with mergers, where quality is measured by mortality, patient safety indicators, readmissions, and complication rates. Studies also find evidence of lower quality in more concentrated hospital markets, both here and abroad. Professor Martin Gaynor, who joins me on this panel today, has published comprehensive analyses of the data and evidence on hospital consolidation and its effects and can speak authoritatively on this body of research.

II.A.2. Physicians

Relative to the acute care hospital industry, there are fewer studies of physician markets. Most analysts subdivide these markets by specific specialties (e.g., cardiology) or groups of specialties (e.g., internists, general practitioners, and family medicine practitioners are often labeled "adult primary care" providers). The geographic market boundaries for services offered by highly-specialized practitioners (e.g., transplant surgeons) are generally larger than the boundaries for services offered by less-specialized practitioners (e.g., pediatricians).

---

[8] These data do not distinguish among the type of hospital (e.g., general acute care, specialty, long-term care, etc.).

[9] Fulton, B. (2017). Health Care Market Concentration Trends in the United States: Evidence and Policy Responses. *Health Affairs,* September 2017, 36:9.

[10] Gaynor, M., Ho, K., and Town, R.J. (2015). The Industrial Organization of Health-Care Markets. *Journal of Economic Literature, 53(2),* 235-284; Vogt, W. & Town, R. (2006). How has hospital consolidation affected the price and quality of hospital care? *Robert Wood Johnson Foundation Synthesis Report* No. 9; Gaynor, M., & Town, R. (2012). The impact of hospital consolidation. *Robert Wood Johnson Foundation Synthesis Report Update.*

There has been a marked increase in the proportion of physicians who are employed rather than owners of their own practices. The rise in employment likely reflects consolidation within physician markets, as most of the investors/employers are hospitals, and the hospital sector is more concentrated than most physician markets. In 1983, 76 percent of physicians reported owning their own practices; this figure stood at 47 percent in 2016.[11]

A recent study of physician markets – defined by specialty and geographic area - finds 22 percent of these markets were highly concentrated, with HHIs in excess of 2,500.[12] This study also found that most changes in physician practice size derived from small acquisitions, characterized as a 'whale eats krill' rather than 'shark eats shark.' The authors observe these acquisitions are generally "too small to trigger Hart-Scott-Rodino notifications and are also too small to be presumptively anticompetitive under the *Horizontal Merger Guidelines.*"

Studies of physician markets find that concentration is associated with higher commercial prices.[13] One such study examined commercially-insured prices for 10 types of office visits in 10 specialties. The researchers found higher price levels and price growth in more concentrated markets.[14]

---

[11] American Medical Association Wire. For first time, physician practice owners are not the majority. Retrieved from https://wire.ama-assn.org/practice-management/first-time-physician-practice-owners-are-not-majority.

[12] Capps, C., Dranove, D., & Ody, C. (2017) Physician Practice Consolidation Driven by Small Acquisitions, So Antitrust Agencies Have Few Tools To Intervene. *Health Affairs.* The authors use a sample of commercial insurance claims data from states accounting for 12 percent of the U.S. population. They define markets for services delivered by 9 specialties to residents in metropolitan statistical areas. Geographic market boundaries are defined so as to satisfy an "outflow" floor of 20 percent, i.e., no more than 20 percent of patients seeking the services of a given specialty seek providers outside the market.

[13] Baker, L.C., Bundorf, M.K., Royalty, A.B., & Levin, Z. (2014). Physician practice competition and prices paid by private insurers for office visits. *JAMA,* 2014:312(16):1653–62; Sun, E., & Baker, L.C. (2015). Concentration in orthopedic markets was associated with a 7 percent increase in physician fees for total knee replacements. *Health Affairs (Millwood);* 34(6):916–21; Dunn, A., Shapiro, A.H. (2014). Do physicians possess market power? *Journal of Law and Economics,* 57(1):159–93.

[14] Baker et al, *ibid.*

II.A.3. Health Insurers

I have written extensively on competition in health insurance markets. My most recent summary of economic evidence on this sector appears in a paper entitled "Evaluating the Impact of Health Insurance Industry Consolidation: Learning from Experience," attached as Exhibit 1 and paraphrased here. The paper documents the high and rising national market shares of the four largest commercial health insurers: the various Blue Cross and Blue Shield affiliates[15] (accounting for an estimated 52 percent of insured lives in 2014); United (13 percent); Aetna (11 percent); and Cigna (6 percent). Between 2006 and 2014, the sum of the market shares for these four insurers (the "four firm concentration ratio") increased from 74 percent to 83 percent. By comparison, the four-firm concentration ratio for the airline industry in 2014 was 62 percent. I also document an increase in the national four-firm concentration ratio for Medicare Advantage plans, from 57 percent in 2007 to 61 percent in 2015.[16]

Studies of insurance consolidation have examined the impact on both insurance premiums (i.e., the "output" side), and on provider prices (i.e., the "input" side). I begin by summarizing the research on the output side. Several studies document lower insurance premiums in areas with more insurers. These studies span a variety of segments, including the public health insurance marketplaces, the large-group market (self-insured and fully insured plans combined), and Medicare Advantage.[17]

---

[15] I group these affiliates together because they have exclusive territory arrangements that impede competition among them, except in a small number of geographic markets.

[16] These national figures do not necessarily reflect the degree of concentration in insurance markets that are relevant to consumers. Many health plans have a significant local, but not national, presence—Kaiser Permanente, Intermountain, and Geisinger among them. Although "Blue Cross and Blue Shield" consists of many separate insurance companies, most areas include only one. The degree of competition in any product and geographic market depends on the market participants and the characteristics of the products they offer. The American Medical Association's annual reports containing detailed market share information for the top two insurers show that concentration is higher within metropolitan statistical areas (MSAs), on average, than in the nation as a whole. Moreover, this concentration appears to be increasing over time.

[17] Sheingold, S., Nguyen, N., & Chappel, A. (2015). Competition and Choice in the Health Insurance Marketplaces, 2014–2015: Impact on Premiums. Washington, D.C.: U.S. Department of Health and Human Services. ASPE Issue Brief. Retrieved from http://aspe.hhs.gov/basic-report/competition-and-choice-health-insurance-marketplaces-2014-2015-impact-premiums; Song, Z., Landrum, M. B., & Chernew, M. E. (2012).

The best available evidence on the impact of insurance consolidation comes from what are known as "event studies" or "merger retrospectives." There are two studies that fall in this category. One, which I coauthored, examines the impacts of a mega-merger in 1999 (Aetna-Prudential) on large-group premiums in 139 distinct geographic markets.[18] We find that premiums increased more in areas with greater pre-merger market overlap. Moreover, the premium increase was not limited to the merging insurers; where the merging firms had substantial overlap, rival insurers raised premiums as well.

A second study examined the impact of the 2008 merger of Sierra Health and UnitedHealth on small-group premiums in two Nevada markets. As compared with control cities in the South and West, small-group premiums in these markets increased by 13.7 percent the year following the merger.[19]

Turning to the research on the relationship between insurance consolidation and input prices, several studies find hospital prices paid on behalf of commercially-insured patients are lower when insurance market concentration is higher. This relationship also holds when researchers study changes over time: in markets that are becoming more concentrated, there is slower growth in hospital prices. Finally, the study of the Aetna-Prudential merger also finds post-merger reductions in wage growth of health care professionals in geographic markets where the merging parties had greater pre-merger overlap. However, if provider price reductions are not ultimately passed through in the form of lower insurance premiums and out-of-pocket payments, they will not benefit consumers. (Even if price

---

Competitive Bidding in Medicare: Who Benefits from Competition? *American Journal of Managed Care*, 18(9):546–52.; Dafny, L., Gruber, J., & Ody, C. (2015). More Insurers, Lower Premiums: Evidence from Initial Pricing in the Health Insurance Marketplaces. *American Journal of Health Economics*, (1):53–81. One recent study suggests premiums for fully-insured employers are lower where insurer concentration is lower, but premiums for self-insured employers are higher; Trish, E. E., & Herring, B.J. (2015). How Do Health Insurer Market Concentration and Bargaining Power with Hospitals Affect Health Insurance Premiums? *Journal of Health Economics*, 42:104–14.

[18] Dafny, L., Duggan, M., & Ramanarayanan, S. (2012). Paying a Premium on Your Premium? Consolidation in the U.S. Health Insurance Industry. *American Economic Review*, 102(2):1161–85.

[19] Guardado et al., *ibid*.

reductions are realized and passed through, if they are achieved as a result of monopsonization of health care markets, consumers may experience an offsetting harm.)

Sections II.A.1 - II.A.3 above highlight consolidation in a select set of health care subsectors. Consolidation is not limited to these sectors, however. There are a number of other subsectors in which consolidation has been documented – ranging from dialysis facilities to generic drug manufacturers to pharmaceutical benefit managers.

II.B. Non-Horizontal Consolidation

There is comparatively little evidence on non-horizontal consolidation, both due to data shortages and to the difficulty in grouping together the myriad types of transactions that fall into this broad category.

Below, I summarize the evidence on the two types of non-horizontal consolidation studied by academic health economists.

II.B.1. "Cross-Market" Hospital Consolidation

Much of the hospital M&A in recent years has occurred across geographies rather than within the same geographic market. Figure 2 below presents data from a study I coauthored on these "cross-market" mergers.[20] The figure shows that of 528 general acute care hospital mergers occurring between 2000 and 2012, more than half did not involve any overlap of the merging parties within the same metropolitan area. More than a third of the transactions involved within-state combinations, and 15 percent involved parties without any hospitals in the same states.

My coauthors and I find that hospitals gaining system members in-state (but not in the same geographic market) experience price increases (for commercially-insured patients) of 7-10 percent relative to a similar group of control hospitals, while hospitals gaining system members out-of-state exhibit no statistically significant changes in price. Another study finds independent hospitals acquired by systems lacking another hospital

---

[20] Dafny, L., Ho, V., & Lee, R. (2017). The Price Effects of Cross-Market Hospital Mergers. *NBER Working Paper* 22106.

within 45 minutes of the target hospital raise the price of the target by 17-18 percent.[21]

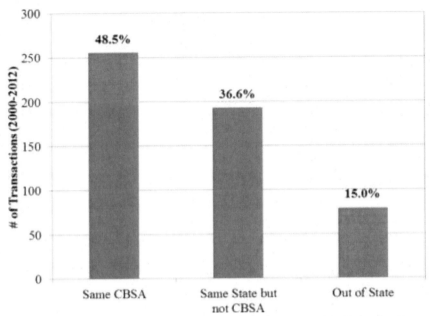

Notes: Based on 528 general acute care hospital mergers reported by Irving Levin over 2000-2012. CBSA= Core-Based Statistical Area.
Source: Dafny, Ho, and Lee (2017). "The Price Effects of Cross-Market Hospital Mergers," NBER Working Paper 22106.

Figure 2. Vertical Chain of Production for Orthopedic Surgery.

Last, a recently published study finds cost reductions among hospitals acquired by an out-of-market system, using a variety of market definitions (e.g., county, or "hospital referral region").[22] Taken together, the research suggests cross-market hospital mergers are profitable endeavors for the merging parties. There is no published research on the effects of cross-market hospital mergers on the quality or range of services offered to patients.

---

[21] Lewis, M.S., and K.E. Pflum. (2016). Hospital Systems and Bargaining Power: Evidence from Out-of-Market Acquisitions. *RAND Journal of Economics* 48(3), 589-610.
[22] Schmitt, M. (2017). Do Hospital Mergers Reduce Costs? *Journal of Health Economics*.

II.B.2. Hospital-Physician Consolidation

Vertical integration of hospitals and physician practices has increased substantially in recent years. For example, one recent study finds that 10 percent of physicians were acquired by a hospital over the period 2007 to 2013, increasing the percentage of physicians in hospital-owned practices by 50 percent.[23] A second study, based on survey data from the AHA also finds an increase of over 50 percent in the market share of fully integrated organizations between 2001 and 2007, from 23 to 36 percent.[24]

A spate of recent studies finds hospital-physician consolidation is followed by price increases for physician services, and in settings where price is fixed (i.e., Medicare), to increases in total spending.[25] There are at least two sources of the spending increases: (1) a shift to "facility-based billing," in which hospital-based providers charge facility and professional fees for outpatient visits – which combined amount to more than the price paid for a physician visit billed independently from a hospital;[26] (2) an increase in prices for these physicians' services following the acquisition of their practices.[27]

---

[23] Capps, C., Dranove, D., & Ody, C. (2015). The Effect of Hospital Acquisitions of Physician Practices on Prices and Spending. *The Institute for Policy Research Northwestern University Working Paper Series.*

[24] *Ibid*, and Baker, L., Bundorf, K., & Kessler, D. (2014). Vertical Integration: Hospital Ownership of Physician Practices is Associated with Higher Prices and Spending. *Health Affairs* 33(5): 756–63.

[25] Neprash, H.T., Chernew, M.E., Hicks, A.L., Gibson, T.,& J.M. McWilliams. (2015). Association of Financial Integration between Physicians and Hospitals with Commercial Health Care Prices. *Journal of the American Medical Association Internal Medicine* 175(12):1932–39; Robinson, J.C., & Miller, K. (2014). Total Expenditures per Patient in Hospital-Owned and Physician-Owned Physician Organizations in California. *Journal of the American Medical Association* 312(16): 1663–69; Koch, T., Wendling, B., & Wilson, N. (2017). How vertical integration affects the quantity and cost of care for Medicare beneficiaries. *Journal of Health Economics.* 52:19-32.

[26] Song, Z., Wallace, J., Neprash, H.T., McKellar, M.R., Chernew, M.E., & McWilliams, J. (2015). Medicare Fee Cuts and Cardiologist-Hospital Integration. *Journal of the American Medical Association Internal Medicine* 175(7): 1229–31.; Dranove, D.,& Ody, C. (2016). Employed for Higher Pay? How Medicare Facility Fees Affect Hospital Employment of Physicians. *Unpublished paper.*

[27] Dranove, D., & Ody, C. (2016). *Ibid.*

Finally, a recent study shows that Medicare's 340b program has led hospitals to increase their employment of physicians in certain specialties, chiefly hematology-oncology, ophthalmology, and rheumatology.[28]

III. The Reasons: Why Consolidation Is Occurring

As compared to the foregoing discussion of consolidation trends and effects – a topic about which there is a substantial body of research available (albeit with significant gaps in certain areas), there is less research attempting to identify motivations for mergers. Thus, what follows is my personal perspective on the likely drivers of consolidation, based on the limited research available, deductive inference, press reports, merger reviews by government agencies, and discussions with industry leaders and commentators.

Fundamentally, what drives consolidation is the expectation it will yield rewards for the merging parties and their stakeholders. I divide these (perceived or actual) rewards into four categories: the ability to reduce competition, scale economies, benefits from insurer reimbursement policies, and care coordination. (A fifth would be empire-building, about which I have little comment but I believe it is a driver.)

As the summary of evidence in the preceding section ("the facts") makes clear, consolidation in various healthcare sectors tends to result in higher commercial prices and/or total spending. Assuming these are profitable decisions, the additional funds gathered as a result can be allocated to profits or to other activities, such as academic research, charity care, or unprofitable service lines (e.g., "margin" or "mission").

Because many healthcare prices are set via negotiation (as opposed to a "posted price" setting, which is common when individual purchasers are responsible for a small share of the seller's business), one key motivation to merge is to gain *bargaining leverage* in negotiations with the relevant counterparty.

---

[28] Desai, S. & McWilliams, J.M., (2018). Consequences of the 340B Drug Pricing Program. *New England Journal of Medicine*, 378:539-548.

Economists have developed and tested formal models of leverage for the case of health care providers; in these models, leverage derives from the added value ("willingness to pay," in the economists' vernacular) that a provider (or a set of merging providers) creates for enrollees of an insurance plan that includes those providers in its network (relative to excluding the provider(s)). Studies of physician and hospital mergers show this leverage is correlated with higher private prices, controlling for a host of other factors affecting price.

When prices are posted, mergers can enable profitable price increases (or reductions in quality that is costly to produce) because purchasers have fewer alternative options. Mergers of insurers selling plans to individuals or to small groups may be motivated in part by the ability to relax competition in their respective markets.

A second driver of mergers appears to be the desire to realize *economies of scale or scope*, that is, lower costs as a result of increased organizational size. Potential sources of scale economies include bulk purchasing discounts, elimination of redundant activities (e.g., billing and collection units or corporate headquarters), and reoptimization or reallocation of activities across sites. Although companies and boards routinely express their expectation that mergers will reduce costs, there is relatively limited evidence to suggest reductions in cost following mergers.[29] Notably, reductions in cost may not be passed through to consumers, and may derive from the (anticompetitive) exercise of monopsony power on the part of the merging buyers.

A third driver of consolidation – particularly hospital-physician transactions – are specific CMS reimbursement policies that increase payments or margins for merged relative to separate entities. As noted above, researchers have shown that the acquisition of physician practices has increased as a result of the higher reimbursement payments available through CMS for hospital-affiliated physicians, a payment practice often

---

[29] I am aware of two studies that have found cost reductions following hospital mergers (Schmitt, previously cited; and Dranove and Lindrooth (1988), and scores of others that have not. I know of no academic research on post-merger cost reductions in other provider settings, or in the health insurance sector.

mimicked by private payers.[30] There is also recent evidence that CMS' reimbursement policies via the 340b program have contributed to an increase in acquisition of specialty practices by hospitals.[31]

A fourth driver of consolidation is the desire to integrate care across multiple organizations. There is little evidence that common ownership produces more integrated care[32] – let alone that this care is better or cheaper than care delivered by affiliations of providers – but merging parties often cite this motive. In addition, shifts in payment models are likely to reward the ability of organizations to generate savings through care coordination, so to the extent that joint ownership facilitates the coordination or is perceived to facilitate it, the desire to coordinate care is another driver of consolidation. That said, one recent study finds consolidation preceded the Affordable Care Act, which established a mechanism for integrated delivery organizations (i.e., Accountable Care Organizations) to reap rewards for integrated care. The authors conclude "little evidence exists" to support the contention that providers have consolidated to participate in "alternative payment models."[33]

IV. The Responses: Current Responses of the Private and Public Sectors to Consolidation

The public-sector response to health care industry consolidation to date largely mirrors the public-sector response to consolidation in other sectors, with some notable exceptions arising from state-specific institutions (e.g.,

---

[30] Dranove, D., & Ody, C. (2016). Employed for Higher Pay? How Medicare Facility Fees Affect Hospital Employment of Physicians. *Unpublished paper;* Song, Z., Wallace, J., Neprash, H.T., McKellar, M.R., Chernew, M.E., & McWilliams, J. (2015). Medicare Fee Cuts and Cardiologist-Hospital Integration. *Journal of the American Medical Association Internal Medicine,* 175(7): 1229–31.
[31] Desai, S. & McWilliams, J.M. (2018). *Ibid.*
[32] Burns, L.R., & Pauly, M. (2012). Accountable Care Organizations May Have Difficulty Avoiding the Failures of Integrated Delivery Networks of the 1990s. *Health Affairs,* 31(11): 2407–15.
[33] Neprash, H.T., Chernew, M.E., & McWilliams, J.M. (2017). Little Evidence Exists To Support The Expectation That Providers Would Consolidate To Enter New Payment Models. *Health Affairs,* 36(2).

state departments of insurance) and legislation pertaining to Certificates of Need and Certificates of Public Advantage.

IV.A. Public Sector Responses

IV.A.1. Antitrust Enforcement

As is the case for other sectors, the federal antitrust enforcement agencies, along with the state attorneys general, investigate potentially anticompetitive mergers and acquisitions. They issue legal complaints to block or dissolve transactions they deem anticompetitive, and then litigate or negotiate consent decrees (i.e., settlements) to address their concerns. The FTC has vigorously pursued provider mergers since conducting its Hospital Merger Retrospectives Analysis in 2002-2004. The Antitrust Division of the Department of Justice has investigated numerous insurer transactions, most recently blocking two mega-mergers (Aetna-Humana and Anthem-Cigna) proposed in 2015. In both cases, federal district courts issued preliminary injunctions to block the transactions, following which the parties abandoned their deals. The healthcare sector is clearly a priority for the federal enforcement agencies, and has been declared as such by their leaders.[34]

As you are aware, the federal antitrust agencies enforce federal antitrust statutes, with Section 7 of the Clayton Act the most relevant for our purposes here. Section 7 prohibits the acquisition of assets or interests where "the effect of such acquisition may be substantially to lessen competition, or to tend to create a monopoly." The statute is narrow, and thus enforcement authorities are not in a position to block all consolidation that may harm consumers. For example, if hospitals acquire physician practices and reap increases in revenues owing to higher payments for services rendered by hospital-affiliated physicians, unless that increase in

---

[34] For example: Ohlhausen, M.K. (2017). The First Wealth is Health: Protecting Competition in Healthcare Markets. *Remarks at the 2017 ABA Fall Forum.* Retrieved from: https://www.ftc.gov/system/files/documents/public_statements/1275573/mko_fall_forum_2 017.pdf.

payment derives from a lessening of competition, Section 7 alone does not provide grounds for antitrust enforcers to challenge the practice.

The way in which Section 7 has been interpreted by federal enforcement authorities has also limited its scope. In particular, Section 7 has largely been interpreted by authorities to require a definition of a relevant antitrust market in which the lessening of competition will occur (or has allegedly occurred) as a result of the transaction. There are many judicial precedents and economic tools used to define relevant antitrust markets, for example the "hypothetical monopolist test," which asserts that a market is not drawn too narrowly if a hypothetical monopolist consisting of all suppliers in the market could profitably raise price by a small, nontrivial amount. However, defining such markets can be challenging in the case of non-horizontal transactions. For example, consider the case of mergers of hospitals across geographic markets. Arguably, these hospitals are rivals to others competing for inclusion in an insurer's network, as insurers are intermediaries between providers and patients, and patients generally face higher prices when utilizing out-of-network providers. Insurer networks typically span a broader geographic area than well-defined acute-care hospital service markets. If the enforcement authorities stipulate the broader insurer boundaries when defining a relevant antitrust market, they may face opposition when proposing narrower markets for horizontal acute-care hospital merger challenges. Recent enforcement successes spearheaded by the Federal Trade Commission (on cases often joined by state authorities) have often relied upon successfully defending these narrow market definitions. Pursuing different or broader market definitions as may be necessary to challenge non-horizontal transactions – is a risky endeavor.

Some state enforcement agencies may be more willing to embrace this challenge and to bear the associated risk. Regardless, enforcement is a blunt and limited instrument for addressing the harms associated with consolidation in the industry to date, and consolidation yet to come.

IV.A.2. State Agencies and Actions

There are a number of state regulations, statutes, and agencies impacting health care consolidation. These include "certificate of need" (CON) laws, "certificate of public advantage" (COPA) laws, state Departments of Insurance, and agencies engaged in monitoring of the health care sector.

Empirical evidence on CON laws – which limit entry and therefore increase the degree of concentration in markets where entrants must seek a CON - finds they are associated with reductions in the quality of regulated services.[35]

COPA laws "allow healthcare providers to enter into cooperative agreements that might otherwise be subject to antitrust scrutiny...[so as] to reduce 'unnecessary' duplication of healthcare resources and control healthcare costs."[36] COPAs have resurged recently and prevented the FTC from pursuing legal challenges in two recent cases: Cabell Huntington-St. Mary's Medical Center (in West Virginia), and Mountain State Health Alliance-Wellmont Health System (in Tennessee and Virginia). In both matters, the FTC testified that the terms of the COPAs are unlikely to produce benefits that outweigh the harms likely to arise from a reduction in competition. In November 2017, the FTC announced its intention to host a public workshop to discuss empirical research on the impact of COPAs.

Both COPAs and CONs substitute regulation for competition, and as such tend to lead to higher industry concentration and consolidation.

States have also reacted to consolidation via their various regulatory bodies. Here, I describe one such body in the Massachusetts, the Massachusetts Health Policy Commission (HPC). The HPC "is charged with developing health policy to reduce overall cost growth while improving the quality of care, and monitoring the health care delivery and

---

[35] Citations are included in recent testimony offered by the Federal Trade Commission before the Alaska Senate. See https://www.ftc.gov/system/files/documents/advocacy_documents/statement-federal-trade-commission-alaska-senate-committee-labor-commerce-certificate-need-laws/p859900_ftc_testimony_before_alaska_senate_re_con_laws.pdf.

[36] FTC Staff Notice of COPA Assessment (2017), retrieved from https://www.ftc.gov/system/files/attachments/press-releases/ftc-staff-seeks-empirical-research-public-comments-regarding-impact-certificates-public-advantage/p181200_copa_assessment_comment_notice_11-1-17.pdf.

payment systems in Massachusetts." It is governed by an 11-person board with a pre-specified set of expertise areas, including health care management, consumer advocacy, primary care, behavioral health, health plan administration, and health economic. Since the HPC was established, Massachusetts' annual per capita spending growth has remained below the national average. All "material ownership changes" must be reported to the Health Policy Commission, which in turn may conduct a "Cost and Market Impact Review" of transactions it deems significant. The HPC may refer transactions generating concern to the Attorney General for further investigation. The process injects substantial transparency into the public debate over the merits of specific mergers, and enables various stakeholders to gain more insight into areas of potential benefit or concern. These stakeholders may use the information reported by the HPC to weigh in on the transactions, and in fact stakeholders have done so in a variety of venues.

IV.B. Private Sector Responses

Setting aside private antitrust challenges and weighing in on specific transactions in public hearings and through meetings with relevant state and federal antitrust officials, the primary tool at the disposal of the private sector is declining to purchase products and services whose prices exceed their perceived or actual value. A comprehensive listing of the factors contributing to muted downstream price sensitivity is beyond the scope of my testimony. Many of these factors are discussed in "Health Care Needs Real Competition," a 2016 article I coauthored (attached as Exhibit 2). In my opinion, one of the central factors impeding an effective private-sector response to anticompetitive mergers in the U.S. is our heavy reliance on employer-sponsored insurance, together with a limited set of options ordinarily offered to employees by employers. U.S. consumers cannot easily select health plans that reflect their preferences over price, network breadth, drug formularies, and so on, so they cannot "vote with their feet."

A second response of private consumers is "forward integration" into the healthcare sector, i.e., choosing to enter the industry rather than to purchase its services. Recent examples include the decision of several hospital systems to enter the generic drug industry, and three large employers to form a joint venture to develop and purchase health care services. These efforts are a clear signal that the healthcare industry is not satisfying the expectations and needs of even the largest buyers.

V. Recommendations: What Else Could Be Done?

The suboptimal performance of the healthcare sector is a critical economic issue, and consolidation in the sector is a contributing factor. I have four specific recommendations for actions that Congress could pursue:

1) Create public databases containing information about the ownership and financial links among different health care providers, and net commercial prices for their services. This database could form the basis for regularly scheduled reports and public hearings on industry consolidation and its effects. I expect that a similar database for prescription drugs that could be of value; I defer to colleagues with greater expertise to weigh in on what data elements ought to be included in such a database.
2) Appropriate sufficient additional funds to the federal enforcement agencies for enforcement-focused research on healthcare consolidation. Enforcement agencies are avid consumers of such research, but they have few resources to devote to pursuing it. As academics have limited time and resources, and different foci (e.g., they may be interested in the harm wreaked by a particular action, not just in whether it violates antitrust statutes), research executed by the enforcement agencies or via grants awarded from the enforcement agencies to impartial researchers could be of substantial value to enforcers.
3) Explore the possibility of dismantling or revising CMS policies that are known to contribute to consolidation, such as higher payments for hospital-affiliated service provision.

4) Provide financial incentives, or impose regulatory requirements, for employers to utilize or develop so-called "private exchanges" where employees can shop for their preferred healthplans and make choices that reflect their own preferences. Data from the public exchanges suggest consumers are more price-sensitive, and more willing to select narrow-network plans, than are employers. These preferences exert pressure on providers and healthplans to develop lower-cost health care solutions, and can therefore reduce the incentive for anticompetitive upstream mergers or practices. If consumers refuse to pay for a higher-priced product that doesn't offer greater value warranting the price premium, the incentive to pursue anticompetitive consolidation will be diminished.

Mr. HARPER. Thank you very much, Dr. Dafny.

The Chair will now recognize Dr. Schulman for the purposes of an opening statement for 5 minutes.

Welcome.

STATEMENT OF KEVIN A. SCHULMAN

Dr. SCHULMAN. Thank you very much. Thank you, Congressman Harper, Ranking Member DeGette, and members of the sub-committee and committee for inviting me to talk with you today.

I would like to address the impact of hospital consolidation on innovation in healthcare markets. We've been talking about this already this morning, and I am going to frame my remarks around two different types of innovation.

One is called organizational innovation, or how firms improve their performance over time, and the second is called disruptive innovation, or how markets evolve over time, and we've talked about both.

First, I would like to discuss a concept called business architecture, or the manner in which firms make decisions that allow them to generate predictable performance over time.

A business architecture is the product of leadership, culture, strategy, and internal organizational controls and processes. The ability of organizations to develop stable business architectures is one of the most revolutionary business concepts of the last century, compared to the chaos of the 19th century.

There is a downside to this construct, however, in that often a business architecture, which is the way we make decisions, leads to a rigidity of business models that can be very difficult to dislodge.

This lens of business architecture is critical to our assessment of healthcare policy related to hospitals. For the last decade, we have pursued an approach of asking hospitals to create new models of care to drive down healthcare costs.

In essence, we have asked them to replace their stable business architectures that have made them successful as fee-for-service providers. This would be a dramatic transformation if any business could achieve this goal.

The business architecture of many hospitals revolves around admitting patients for treatment, especially patients with commercial insurance or those who require surgery.

The hospital is treated as a profit center. In other words, the more the service is provided, the better financially for the system.

In these models, providers and hospital networks exist to provide patient referrals for inpatient care. Hospital mergers extend this model by making clinical services even more costly in multihospital systems.

To better understand the rigidity of the hospital business architecture, we asked a sample of chief financial officers about their planning for business transformation. We wanted to understand what types of investments would be required to pivot from a fee for service business model to the most extreme value-based payment model capitation.

We found that none of the leaders we interviewed had a clear estimate of the investment that would be required for the same transformation and observed in the crosshair sample there significant disagreements about how a change in payment models would impact essential components of the budget models.

Despite almost a decade to prepare for this transformation, there is little evidence of the development of the concrete business plans that would be required to successfully carry out business architecture change.

One approach to organizational change is to create a new leadership role tasked with innovation—a chief innovation officer. These leaders could help guide the transformation of the delivery system to new models of care that we all desire.

Eighty percent of the largest health systems in the United States have created such a role, and we surveyed a majority of these individuals. While the respondents were all enthusiastic and committed to innovation, we were very concerned after this research. These roles were not structured or budgeted for success.

For example, when these respondents reported that their role was strategic—in other words, that they were responsible for this change—their median annual budget was only $3 million. It's unlikely that investments of this magnitude can change business architectures within these enormous, multibillion-dollar organizations.

Large hospital systems can have other impacts on innovation. Vertically integrated organizations are good at developing standard business processes but are not necessarily conducive to the type of physician-driven innovation that could drive new care models.

In part, this concern could explain why there's little evidence of the quality of care improving when hospitals pursue physician employment models.

One way to reconcile these findings is to realize that, rather than pursue business transformation that we have been seeking, hospitals have been actively pursuing an agenda related to market power. The impacts of market power on business strategy and hospital investments can have sustained impact over long periods of time.

The other type of innovation I would like to discuss is disruptive innovation, or changes in business models within markets. Clay Christensen has described how technology innovation allows business innovation to bring about cost and quality improvements for consumers.

At the core, Christensen suggests that business architecture of existing firms is so rigid that they can't respond to market changes that they plainly see and so are replaced by new entrants in a process of created destruction within markets.

Hospital-led organizations are the type of large, inefficient firms theory suggests should be replaced. If you wake up with a sore throat, would you rather go to a hospital and pay for parking, wait to be seen, or just have a telemedicine consult to tell you whether or not you need antibiotics?

The lack of disruptive innovation is a critical shortfall in the healthcare market. Not only could disruptive innovation drive development of novel clinical services for patients, but would shake up the market to spur existing hospitals to more fully embrace an innovation agenda.

One recent study suggested that 50 percent of the increase in healthcare costs since 1996 is related to service and price intensity. This is the pattern of costs that would be expected to result from the migration of clinical services to the hospital-based business model with all of this consolidation.

Overall, all of this is a tremendous price for American consumers to pay for the failure of an innovation agenda in healthcare.

Thank you.

[The statement of Dr. Schulman follows:]

TESTIMONY, KEVIN A. SCHULMAN, MD, PROFESSOR OF MEDICINE DUKE UNIVERSITY DURHAM, NC, VISITING SCHOLAR HARVARD BUSINESS SCHOOL, BOSTON, MA, COMMITTEE ON ENERGY AND COMMERCE SUBCOMMITTEE ON OVERSIGHT AND INVESTIGATIONS, FEBRUARY 14, 2018

Summary Points

- Firms have a business architecture that is a product of leadership, culture and internal controls. Business architectures can lead to a rigidity of business models that is difficult to change.
- The business architecture of many hospitals often revolves around admitting patients for treatment, where financial performance is directly related to the volume of services.
- Innovation can extend to asking hospitals to change their business architecture (organizational innovation), or fostering entry of new business models that replace hospital-centric delivery systems (disruptive innovation).
- In our work, we have documented the limited degree to which hospitals are preparing for a transformation in their business architecture.
- In this analysis, hospital consolidation is often an extension of the current business architecture, and may provide a barrier to novel business models in the market.
- Disruptive innovation offers a model for transformation of care models that offer lower cost and higher quality over time. There is little evidence that large fee-for-service hospital systems are embracing these types of approaches as a replacement for their current business architectures.
- One recent study suggested that 50% of the increase in health care costs since 1996 is related to service price and intensity, a pattern

that would be expected from the migration of clinical services to the hospital-based business model. Overall, this is the tremendous price American consumers are paying for the failure of an innovation agenda in health care.

Thank you, Congressman Harper and members of the Committee for inviting me to speak with you.

I'm joined on this panel by two esteemed health economists who have conducted much of the research describing the impact of hospital consolidation on health care costs in this country. It is hard to argue with their findings and I want to applaud their careful methodologic work on this topic.

Today, I would like to address the impact of hospital consolidation on innovation in the health care markets. Specifically, I will address both organizational innovation, or how firms evolve, and disruptive innovation, or how markets evolve.

First, I'd like to discuss a concept called business architecture, or the manner in which firms make decisions that allow them to generate predictable performance over time. A business architecture is a product of leadership, culture and internal organizational controls. The ability to develop a stable business architecture is one of the most revolutionary business concepts of the last century. There is a downside to this construct, however, in that often the business architecture leads to a rigidity of business models that is difficult to dislodge.

I believe that the lens of business architecture is critical to our assessment of health care policy related to hospitals. For the last decade, we have pursued a policy approach of asking hospitals to create new models of care to drive down health care costs. In essence, we have asked them to change the stable business architectures that have made them successful in a fee-for-service business model, to define a new business architecture.[37] This would be a dramatic transformation if it was achieved.

---

[37] Richman BD, Mitchell W, Schulman KA. Organizational innovation in health care. *Health Management, Policy and Innovation*. 2013;1(3):36-44.

The business architecture of many hospitals often revolves around admitting patients for treatment, especially patients with commercial insurance or patients who require a test or surgical procedure. The hospital is treated as a profit-center within the system. In other words, the more hospital services provided the better financially for the system. In these models, provider and hospital networks seem to exist to provide patient referrals for inpatient care.

Hospital mergers extend this model by making clinical services even more costly in multi-hospital systems.[38]

To better understand the rigidity of the hospital business architecture, we asked a small sample of Chief Financial Officers of academic medical centers about their planning for this transformation. Specifically, we wanted to understand what types of investments were required to pivot from a fee-for-service business model to the most extreme value-based payment model, capitation. We found that none of the leaders we interviewed had a clear estimate of the investment required for this transformation, and observed that across our sample that there were significant disagreements about how such a transformation in payment models would impact essential components of their budget models.[39] In our interpretation, despite almost a decade to prepare for this transformation, there was little evidence of development of the concrete business planning that would be required to successfully carry out business architecture change.

One approach to organizational change is to create a new leadership role tasked with innovation, in many cases a Chief Innovation Officer (CInO). In principle, these leaders could help guide the transformation of these multi-billion-dollar delivery systems to new models of care. Eighty percent of the largest health systems in the US have created such a role, and we surveyed the majority of these individuals. While the respondents were all enthusiastic and committed to innovation, we were very concerned that these roles were not structured or budgeted for success. For example,

---

[38] Robinson JC, Miller K. Total expenditures per patient in hospital-owned and physician-owned physician organizations in California. JAMA. 2014 Oct 22-29;312(16):1663-9.

[39] Poku M, Schulman KA. We Interviewed Industry Leaders About Their Industry and They're Worried. Harvard Business Review. December 14, 2016.

when the respondents reported that their role was strategic (rather than operational or financial), their median annual budget was only $3 million.[40] Such investments are unlikely to drive significant change in business architectures within large organizations.

Large hospital systems can have other impacts on innovation. In our analysis of the literature, we were very concerned that vertically integrated organizations were good at developing standard business processes, but were not conducive to the type of physician-driven innovation that could enable new care models.[41] In part, this concern could explain why there is little evidence that the quality of health care improves when hospitals pursue physician employment models.[42]

One way to reconcile these findings is to realize that rather than pursue the business transformation we seek, hospitals have been actively pursuing an agenda related to market power. The impacts of market power on business strategy and hospital investments can have sustained effects over long periods of time.[43]

The other type of innovation I would like to discuss is disruptive innovation, or changes in business models within markets. We have seen wholesale changes in business models in many markets in the US and globally, all enabled by the tremendous changes in information technology over the last few decades. Clay Christensen has described how technology innovation allows business model innovation to bring about cost and quality improvements for consumers.[44]

---

[40] Sneha P. Shah, MBA; Lauren McCourt, BA, BS; Kristina Jakobson, BA; Amy Saddington, BS; Kate Harvey, MBA; Kevin A. Schulman, MD. Leading Change—A National Survey of Chief Innovation Officers in Health Systems. Health Management, Policy and Innovation, 2018. www.hmpi.org. (pre-publication draft attached).

[41] Huesch MD, Schulman KA, Douglas PS. Could accountable care organizations stifle physician learning and innovation? *Health Management, Policy and Innovation*. 2014;2(1):18-28.

[42] Kirstin W. Scott, MPhil, PhD; E. John Orav, PhD; David M. Cutler, PhD; Ashish K. Jha, MD, MPH. Changes in Hospital–Physician Affiliations in U.S. Hospitals and Their Effect on Quality of Care. Ann Intern Med. 2017;166(1):1-8.

[43] Robinson J. Hospitals Respond To Medicare Payment Shortfalls By Both Shifting Costs And Cutting Them, Based On Market Concentration. Health Aff (Millwood). 2011 Jul;30(7):1265-71.

[44] Christensen CM. The Innovator's Dilemma: When New Technologies Cause Great Firms to Fail. Harvard Business Review Press. 1997.

At the core, Christensen suggests that often the business architecture of existing firms is so rigid that they cannot respond to the market changes that they plainly see, and so they are replaced by new entrants. This cycle of creative destruction of firms is responsible for the remarkable changes we have seen in the technology markets.

Hospital-led organizations are the types of large, inefficient firms that this theory suggests should be replaced in the market by new business models. Would you rather go to your physician's office, pay to park by the hour, wait in a waiting room to be seen for 15 minutes, and then find out you don't need a prescription after you have lost two hours away from work, or would you prefer to just receive a Telemedicine consult to determine whether your symptoms are those of a virus requiring treatment with hot tea or those of a strep throat requiring confirmation and antibiotics? There is little evidence that large fee-for-service hospital systems are embracing these types of approaches as a replacement for their current business architectures.

The lack of disruptive innovation is a critical shortfall in the healthcare market. Not only could disruptive innovation drive development of novel clinical services for patients, emphasizing care at the lowest possible cost (generally far away from the hospital), but it could also serve as a significant catalyst to spur existing hospitals and systems within a market to more fully embrace an innovation agenda.

This lack of innovation in the business architecture of health care firms has an enormous cost for all of us. It is no secret that health care costs have increased by 56% since 2008.[45] One recent study suggested that 50% of the increase in health care costs since 1996 is related to service price and intensity,[46] a pattern that would be expected from the migration of clinical services to the hospital-based business model. In 2017, employer and employee contributions for health insurance reached $18,764 per

---

[45] Centers for Medicair and Medicaid Services. NHE Projections. https://www.cms.gov/research-statistics-data-and-systems/statistics-trends-and-reports/nationalhealthexpenddata/national healthaccountsprojected.html. Accessed on February 4, 2018.
[46] Joseph L. Dieleman, PhD[1]; Ellen Squires, MPH[1]; Anthony L. Bui, MPH[2]; et al. Factors Associated With Increases in US Health Care Spending, 1996-2013. *JAMA*. 2017;318(17):1668-1678.

household,[47] with employee contributions rising 270% since 1999.12 Moreover, these escalating costs are found despite a significant shift to less generous benefit designs such as high-deductible health plans (now 28% of the health insurance market[48]).

Overall, this is the tremendous price American consumers are paying for the failure of an innovation agenda in health care.

LEADING CHANGE—A NATIONAL SURVEY OF CHIEF INNOVATION OFFICERS IN HEALTH SYSTEMS

Sneha P. Shah, MBA; Lauren McCourt, BA, BS; Kristina Jakobson, BA; Amy Saddington, BS; Kate Harvey, MBA; Kevin A. Schulman*, MD

Author Affiliations: Harvard Business School, Boston, Massachusetts (Ms Shah); Russell Reynolds Associates, New York, New York (Mss McCourt, Jakobson, Saddington, and Harvey); and Duke Clinical Research Institute and Department of Medicine, Duke University School of Medicine, Durham, North Carolina (Dr Schulman)

*Corresponding Author: Kevin A. Schulman, Duke Clinical Research Institute, PO Box 17969, Durham, NC 27715; telephone: 919-668-8101; kevin.schulman@duke.edu.

Forthcoming: Health Management, Policy and Innovation (www.HMPI.Org)

2686 words

Survey of Chief Innovation Officers, October 2, 2017

---

[47] The Henry J. Kaiser Family Foundation. 2017 Employer Health Benefits Survey. https://www.kff.org/health-costs/report/2017-employer-health-benefits-survey/. Accessed on January 30, 2018.

[48] The Henry J. Kaiser Family Foundation. Employer Health Benefits Survey 2017. http://files.kff.org/attachment/Release-Slides-2017-Employer-Health-Benefits-Survey. Accessed on January 30, 2018.

Abstract

Importance: Health care organizations are developing chief innovation officer roles in response to changes in the health care environment.

Objective: To examine the charge, structure, and function of chief innovation officer roles in health care systems.

Design, Setting, and Participants: Structured survey of leaders at the 40 largest health care systems by revenue in the United States.

Main Outcomes and Measures: Organizational structure, outcomes and metrics, resources, career preparation, and background of individuals in chief innovation officer roles.

Results: Of the 40 largest health care systems in the United States, 32 had a senior innovation officer. Half of respondents (52%) characterized their role as strategic, 24% as operational, and 24% as financial. Structurally, 80% resided within established organizational structures, and 36% reported directly to the chief executive officer. Overall, 44% had short-term metrics of success, 68% medium-term, and 24% long-term (nonexclusive responses). The median budget for the role was $3.5 million, but some organizations invested significantly more, usually in a venture capital function.

Conclusions and Relevance: Chief innovation officer roles have been established in many health systems to guide innovation efforts. Respondents to our survey were enthusiastic, informed, and satisfied with the progress they have been able to make to date. However, whether organizational support and structure around this effort is yet sufficient for transformative innovation of delivery systems towards new models of care is an open question.

Introduction

Health care policy is increasingly designed to incentivize the transformation of health care delivery [1, 2]. Payment model reform requires health systems to develop the capacity to innovate so that they may successfully navigate clinical and organizational transitions to new models of care [3-9]. This shift in focus has led to the rise of an "innovation agenda" in health care [10-12]. One of the most visible responses to this agenda has been the rise of "chief innovation officers" in the highest ranks of executive leadership in health systems. The term *chief innovation officer* was described in 1998 as part of a growing recognition that innovation within organizations needed to include continuous and discontinuous, or disruptive, strategies [13]. Individuals in the chief innovation officer roles were to identify new ideas, concepts, and business opportunities, and then develop the capabilities to support and implement this agenda [13].

A PubMed search found that, in 2016, 646 articles had been published on the topic of organizational innovation. However, only 2 articles pertained to the position or mission of chief innovation officers in health care [14, 15]. Both reports were single-institution descriptions of innovation efforts. While more systems are adopting a chief innovation officer as a member of their senior leadership team, little is known about the charge, evaluation, and support of the individuals in these roles.

We sought to better understand the organizational framework, reporting structure, resource allocation, and metrics of success for chief innovation officers. Based on these findings, we can better understand how these roles are structured within health care systems. These data can also allow us use concepts from organizational innovation theory to analyze whether health systems are adequately supporting their chief innovation officers for success of the innovation agenda in health care.

Methods

Survey Development

We developed a survey based on the conceptualized role of the chief innovation officer in health systems using teachings from organizational innovation theory [10-13, 16, 17]. We advanced and tailored these concepts using a set of position specifications available to Russell Reynolds Associates, an executive search firm. Finally, we refined the survey through qualitative interviews with 3 chief innovation officers who volunteered to both respond to the survey and to provide feedback on the survey instrument. The final instrument was designed to be interviewer-administered, prompted by a set of open-ended discussion questions and recorded on a data collection form that included 23 structured questions: 8 questions about organizational charge and structure, 4 about outcomes/metrics, 2 about barriers, 3 about resources, and 4 about career preparation and background. Finally, we developed 2 summary assessment questions, each using a 7-point Likert scale to better characterize the role of the chief innovation officer. The questions were anchored as internally focused vs. commercially focused, and as tactical vs strategic. The survey was considered exempt research by the institutional review board of Harvard University.

Survey Sample

We identified the 40 largest health systems by revenue in the United States using the Definitive Healthcare data set as candidates for our sample. We then used LinkedIn, organization websites, publically available press-releases, and Russell Reynolds Associates' proprietary database to identify the chief innovation officer or most senior innovation-responsible executive at each organization. For organizations where we could not identify a chief innovation through the above methodology, or in the case that the identified chief innovation officer was the wrong executive, we conducted sourcing interviews with industry experts to identify the chief innovation officer or to confirm that the organization had such as position.

Survey Administration

Between January and May 2017, chief innovation officers received an email, consent form, and interview agenda detailing the content of the interview. Interviewers were cross-trained during the month of January to ensure standardization of interview delivery, and interviews were recorded to ensure quality control. Phone interviews were conducted over WebEx, and recordings were stored securely. Each call was attended by 2 interviewers—1 who conducted the interview and the other who took notes during the call.

Nonrespondents received 2 follow-up emails sent 1 week apart, followed by 1 phone call 1 week later. Nonrespondents were contacted once more at 1 month after the initial 4 attempts at outreach. No financial incentive was included to encourage participation, and participants were informed that all data would be deidentified in reporting.

Data Analysis

We developed descriptive statistics for the 23 structured questions derived from the open-ended interview questions. We further categorized these roles using our own categorization of the chief innovation officer role from the qualitative interviews. Data from the structured interviews, the qualitative interviews, and the summary assessment questions are shown graphically in a 2-by-2 figure.

Results

We were unable to identify a chief innovation officer or equivalent position for 8 of the 40 health systems in the sample. This resulted in a sample of 32 organizations with a chief innovation officer or other senior innovation-responsible executive. We were able to complete 25 interviews from this sample, for a response rate of 78%. Of the 25 individuals interviewed, 22 had "innovation" in their title, such as "chief innovation officer" or "senior vice president of strategy and innovation." Nine of these 22 participants had "chief innovation officer" specifically in their title. Three participants did not have "innovation" in their job title but did have the term in their job description, such as "senior vice president of ventures" or "vice president of market development and incubations," and were identified as the senior-most executive charged with the innovation agenda at their health system.

When asked to select whether the primary focus of their role was strategic, operational, or financial, we found that the majority (52%) of participants reported having a strategic focus, 24% operational, and 24% financial (Table 1). In qualitative analysis, we were able to characterize participants' roles into 1 of 4 patterns: (1) an "internal consulting group" that educated, advised, and partnered around continuous process improvement (36%); (2) an incubator that worked to grow and scale projects (28%); (3) a group that imported and scaled established technology (12%); and (4) a venture fund that invested externally and sometimes internally (24%) (Table 2).

In terms of reporting structure, only 36% of participants reported that they reported to the chief executive officer, with 8% reporting to the chief operating office and the rest to other senior leaders of the organization. Table 1 shows the organizational structure by primary focus.

Overall, 72% of participants reported that the organizational board is involved with the innovation efforts of the chief innovation officer. Most often, the board was noted to play an instrumental role in setting up the position or innovation centers in the health system. Subsequently, chief innovation officers often provided the board with quarterly or annual updates, but the board did not play an active role in setting the innovation agenda.

The majority of respondents reported that the innovation function resided within the traditional organizational structure, with 52% reporting that the innovation group is a new business unit within the existing structure, and 28% reporting that the innovation group is an existing business unit within an existing structure. Twelve percent of respondents reported that the innovation group was a new business unit outside of the existing organizational structure, and 8% of respondents reported that the innovation group is a new initiative outside of the traditional structure entirely, such as an external venture capital fund.

Most respondents (72%) reported that their organizations had developed an innovation center of some kind, and 89% of respondents in systems with innovation centers work directly with these centers. Thirty-six percent of respondents reported that they worked with the technology transfer function within their organization, and 72% work with external entrepreneurs, 56% with external venture capital firms, and 32% with external consultants. Sixty-eight percent reported that they have introduced tech solutions as part of their innovation agenda.

We obtained organizational timelines for 24 of the 25 chief innovation officer positions. The median number of years the position has existed at these institutions is 4 years (mean, 5.3 years); 16 (67%) have existed for 5 years or less, 7 (29%) for 6 to 10 years, and 1 (4%) for longer than 10 years.

We asked respondents about metrics used to assess the success of the chief innovation officer function, and 44% reported that the metrics used are short-term, 68% medium-term (1 to 3 years), and 24% long-term (multiple responses were permitted). Metrics reported by participants included individual project measures, counts of outside company partnerships, counts of employees that were influenced or reached, quality metrics, and financial return on investment metrics.

In terms of barriers to innovation, 64% of respondents reported that the biggest barrier is culture or organizational structure, and an equal number of respondents (16%) reported budget, talent, and process as the largest hindrances to innovation. More than 1 response was allowed for this question. Overall, 28% of respondents reported that they spend a disproportionate amount of time advancing the innovation agenda at the executive level of the organization, 36% with operational leadership, 24% with financial leadership, and 24% with clinical or university leadership. None of the respondents reported that they spent a disproportionate amount of time with their board of directors.

Of all respondents, 20 (80%) provided their total budget amount and 24 (96%) shared their headcount. Overall, the median budget under the control of the chief innovation officer in was $3.5 million. There was a strongly skewed distribution of responses; 60% of respondents have a budget of $5 million or less, 15% greater than $5 million but less than or equal to $20 million, and 25% greater than $20 million. The latter group consisted of organizations that have developed their own venture capital funds. The median headcount was 9.5 people; 54% have a headcount of 10 or less, 29% have a headcount less than or equal to 50, and 17% have a headcount greater than 50. Of groups with greater than 50 full-time employees, 75% were organizations with their own venture capital funds. Overall, 68% of respondents reported that they are funded through operational funds, 24% through executive discretionary funds, and the rest through either investment or strategic funds.

In terms of career trajectory, 60% of respondents were internal candidates when appointed. Overall, 44% of respondents reported that they have an MD degree (and of these 45% are still practicing medicine), and 4 of 25 respondents were women.

The results of our summary questions sorted by the charge of the position are shown in the Figure. Overall, chief innovation officer roles that were characterized as strategic were most frequently identified as strategic and internally focused, roles that were characterized as operational were most frequently internally focused, and organizations with a financial charge were most frequently strategic.

Discussion

This study provides important data on the status of the innovation agenda across the largest health care systems. To our knowledge, it is the first study of innovation to look across multiple health systems and to specifically address the role of the chief innovation officer. In response to calls for organizational change, most of the largest health systems established a new leader in their organization to fill the role of a senior innovation officer. The structure and function of the role was be remarkably diverse across systems, in mandate, structure, and budget.

We found a varied set of responses to the definition of innovation within an organization that often tracked with the definition of the chief innovation officer role. The responses reflected thoughtful approaches to the challenges of organizational innovation. As one respondent reflected, the role was created "in recognition that the tyranny of the daily trumps the pursuit of the remarkable...absent a countervailing force....there is a large amount of untapped creative energy in the organization; and it needs a beacon to light the way." This supports findings from the innovation literature: "Most companies have plenty of creativity and plenty of technology. What they lack are the managerial skills to convert ideas into impact" [16].

Innovation can be characterized on a spectrum that includes execution, improvement, and transformation [17]. Execution is focused on ensuring evidence-based practices (such as hand washing). Improvement (also known as sustaining innovation) is focused on incremental betterment of existing processes, products, or services. Transformation (also known as disruptive innovation) is focused on development of novel processes, products, or services that represent a fundamental shift in an approach that will eventually overtake existing processes [14, 15]. All of the participants we interviewed reported that they were focused on improvement or transformation as their core assignment.

The innovation literature has a growing focus on the role of organizational structure as a key enabling approach for organizations to consider, particularly for business transformation [4]. This focus follows from the description of a classic organizational design at Hewlett-Packard's printer division [12], through the restructuring of Google into Alphabet [18]. Yet, in our study, only 20% of respondents reported that innovation included a novel organizational form. This result stands in contrast to an aspiration for transformative innovation in organizations, such as a shift to value-based payment models in health care. This result may limit the impact of these innovation efforts: "When innovators stop short of business model innovation, hoping that a new technology will achieve transformative results without a corresponding disruptive business model and without embedding it in a new disruptive value network or ecosystem, fundamental change rarely occurs" [12].

For most organizations, the chief innovation officer role was characterized as a strategic one. Yet, in only a minority of organizations did the chief innovation officer report to the chief executive. As stated by 1 respondent, "The reporting relationship is critical. [When asked], 'Who owns innovation?,' [our CEO] immediately said, without skipping a beat, 'the CEO does,' even with me sitting next to him. He is absolutely right. If the CEO doesn't own innovation, the organization will eat it alive. It's just not a fair fight. The CEO has to own it, drive it, and value it."

Organizational culture and structure was the category respondents described as the biggest obstacle to success. The most important role of any leader is to establish and communicate a clear vision for the organization. In an organization as complex as a health care system, this is a difficult challenge, even when the market and policy environment is stable.

While conceptually there is an understanding of the transition to value as a payment model in health care, in most markets and policy discussions this remains an aspiration rather than a market imperative. Thus, leaders discuss and address innovation often in the context of supporting existing fee-for-service business models. This lack of clarity at an organizational level can lead to confusion at an operational level in terms of the innovation agenda. As one of our respondents said, "Decide if you want to really innovate or not. Don't pretend. Because that has implications across staffing, funding, organizational commitment."

Most large health care organizations have finely tuned budget models with clear metrics to guide investment decisions. The innovation agenda can be challenging in this type of environment, as by definition innovation is not designed to be predicable and is inherently risky. In addition to investment in new organizational forms, innovation can replace existing legacy business models, such as facilities and clinical or administrative structures. Addressing these legacy issues requires political capital and close-out funding that can be equally difficult to manage from a resource allocation perspective [11]. For most of the organizations in our survey, the chief innovation officer has a modest budget and headcount, given the strategic nature of the role.

Our study is based on self-report by survey respondents. We did not audit the data. When respondent organizations identified a senior leader who was the head of innovation, only 9 had the explicit title of chief innovation officer, and the research team had to determine whether the role was really a senior innovation role.

Chief innovation officer roles have been established in many health systems to guide innovation efforts in response to policy changes in health care. Respondents to our survey were enthusiastic, informed, and satisfied with the progress they have been able to make to date.

However, whether organizational support and structure around this effort is yet sufficient for transformative innovation of delivery systems toward new models of care is an open question.

Acknowledgments

Funding/Support: This work was supported internally by the Duke Clinical Research Institute.

Additional Contributions: Damon M. Seils, MA, Duke University, assisted with manuscript preparation. Mr Seils did not receive compensation for his assistance apart from his employment at the institution where the study was conducted.

REFERENCES

[1] Berwick DM, Hackbarth AD. Eliminating waste in US health care. *JAMA*. 2012;307(14):1513-1516.

[2] Rajkumar R, Press MJ, Conway PH. The CMS Innovation Center-a five-year self-assessment. *N Engl J Med*. 2015;372(21):1981-1983.

[3] McGlynn EA, McClellan M. Strategies for assessing delivery system innovations. *Health Aff* (Millwood). 2017;36(3):408-416.

[4] Ellner AL, Stout S, Sullivan EE, Griffiths EP, Mountjoy A, Phillips RS. Health systems innovation at academic health centers: leading in a new era of health care delivery. *Acad Med*. 2015;90(7):872-880.

[5] Schulman KA, Richman BD. Reassessing ACOs and health care reform. *JAMA*. 2016;316(7):707-708.

[6] Song Z, Fisher ES. The ACO experiment in infancy--looking back and looking forward. *JAMA*. 2016;316(7):705-706.

[7] Poku M, Schulman KA. We interviewed health care leaders about their industry, and they're worried. Harvard Business Review. December 14, 2016. https://hbr.org/2016/12/we-interviewed-health-care-leaders-about-their-industry-and-theyre-worried. Accessed September 13, 2017.

[8] Herzlinger RE, Schleicher SM, Mullangi S. Health care delivery innovations that integrate care? Yes! But integrating what? *JAMA*. 2016;315(11):1109-1110.

[9] Rudin RS, Bates DW, MacRae C. Accelerating innovation in health IT. *N Engl J Med*. 2016;375(9):815-7.

[10] Herzlinger RA, Schulman KA. Diffusions of global innovations in health care: how to make it happen. Health Management, Policy and Innovation 2016;2. http://hmpi.org/2016/10/17/diffusion-of-global-innovations-in-health-care-how-to-make-it-happen/. September 13, 2017.

[11] Richman BD, Mitchell W, Schulman KA. Organizational innovation in health care. *Health Management, Policy and Innovation*. 2013;1(3):36-44.

[12] Christensen CM, Grossman JH, Hwang J. *The Innovator's Prescription: A disruptive Solution for Health Care*. New York: McGraw-Hill; 2009.

[13] Miller W, Morris L. Fourth Generation R&D: Managing Knowledge, Technology, and Innovation. New York: John Wiley & Sons; 1998.

[14] Dulin MF, Lovin CA, Wright JA. Bring big data to the forefront of healthcare delivery: the experience of Carolinas Health Care System. *Front Health Serv Manag*. 2017;33(1):1-12.

[15] Samet K, Smith M. Thinking differently: catalyzing innovation in healthcare and beyond. *Front Health Serv Manag*. 2016;33(2):3-15.

[16] Gobindarajan V, Trimble C. *The Other Side of Innovation: Solving the Execution Challenge*. Boston: Harvard Business Review Press; 2010.

[17] Christenson CM. *The Innovator's Dilemma: When New Technologies Cause Great Firms to Fail*. Boston, MA: Harvard Business School Press; 1997.

[18] Page L. G is for Google. https://googleblog.blogspot.com/2015/08/google-alphabet.html. Accessed September 12, 2017.

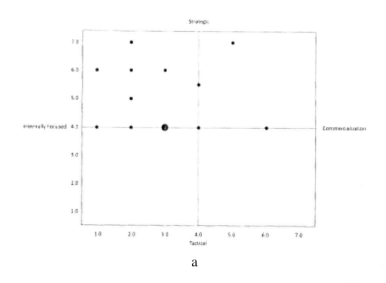

a

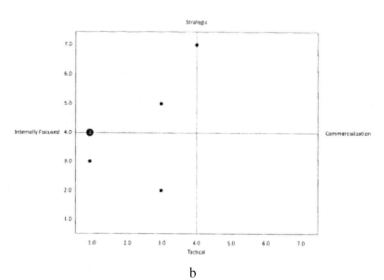

b

Examining the Impact of Healthcare Consolidation ...

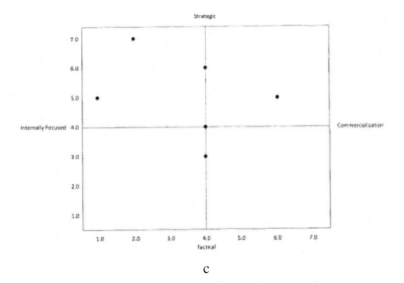

C

Figure. Summary Assessment Questions for Chief Innovation Officers With a Stated Primary Focus That Was Strategic (Panel A), Operational (Panel B), and Financial (Panel C).

Chief innovation officer roles that were characterized as strategic were most frequently identified as strategic and internally focused; roles characterized as operational were most frequently internally focused; and roles with a financial charge were most frequently strategic.

Table 1. Characteristics of chief innovation officers by primary function

Characteristic	Strategic (n = 13)	Operational (n = 6)	Financial (n = 6)	Total (N =25)
Reporting directly to chief executive officer, %	54	0	33	36
Business unit outside existing structures, %	8	0	67	20
Budget (in millions), median, $[a]	3.0	2.0	35.0	3.5
Headcount, median, No.[b]	17.0	6.5	30.0	9.5

[a]Budget data were provided by 9 of 13 chief innovations officers in the strategic function, 5 of 6 in the operational function, and 6 of 6 in the financial function.

[b]Headcount data were provided by 13 of 13 chief innovation officers in the strategic function, 6 of 6 in the operational function, and 5 of 6 in the financial function.

Table 2. Primary stated focus vs. functional categorization of chief innovation officers

Focus	Strategic (n = 13)	Operational (n = 6)	Financial (n = 6)	Total (N =25)
Internal consultants	7/13 (54%)	2/6 (33%)	0	9/25 (36%)
Incubator	5/13 (38%)	2/6 (33%)	0	7/25 (28%)
Import and scale	1/13 (8%)	0	0	3/25 (12%)
Venture	0	0	6/6 (100%)	6/25 (24%)

Mr. HARPER. Thank you, Dr. Schulman, and thanks to each of you for the summary of your testimony.

It's now time for the Members to ask questions. Each Member will have 5 minutes, and as Chair I will recognize myself for 5 minutes and begin.

And I will start with you, Dr. Gaynor, if I may. As you have heard today, obviously, the cost of healthcare has steadily risen over the past several decades, and one of the factors that certainly we are looking at that's contributing are the number of consolidations that have occurred in the healthcare industry the past decade.

So my two questions for you, Dr. Gaynor: What impact has consolidation had on patient cost, quality of care, and access to care, and are there any indications to you that patients are better off after consolidation or with that?

Dr. GAYNOR. Thank you, Chairman Harper.

So the research evidence shows very clearly that consolidations between hospitals that are close competitors lead to very substantial price increases. Depending on the exact situations, it could be as high as 50 percent but not all.

For insurers, again, there's extensive evidence that consolidation among insurers leads to higher premiums, and for physician practices, again, consolidation between physician practices that are close competitors lead to higher prices, in some cases substantial. And last, the acquisitions of physician practices by hospitals lead to higher prices for physician services and more spending.

The evidence on the quality of care, I would say, is mixed. But overall it does not show gains for patients in terms of quality of care.

If anything, there is some evidence that shows that clinical quality of care for patients can suffer when there's less competition between hospitals or doctors, and we do not see, again, consistent evidence of more coordination of care or lower costs of care.

So this harms patients, first, because the costs of care are higher. As we know, that when the costs of care get higher, employers pay higher fringe benefit costs, and those get shifted back onto workers in the form of lower total compensation, whether it's lower wages, paying more out of pocket for health insurance or having less generous health insurance. The average American household hasn't seen an increase in their real standard of living—that of healthcare costs—in quite some time.

So it doesn't appear on average that there are benefits that are being realized, and there are real costs.

Mr. HARPER. Thank you.

And Dr. Dafny, should we be concerned about the increased numbers of consolidation in the healthcare industry?

Dr. DAFNY. Chairman Harper, thank you for the question.

Given the data that Professor Gaynor has just described and that is described in our testimony, I would indeed be concerned, on average.

I keep adding the "on average" because every consolidation needs to be considered on its merits, and there are a number of consolidations that are occurring right now that are pretty novel and I wouldn't propose that those be quashed just because on average consolidation hasn't——

Mr. HARPER. Sure. So you can point to some successful outcomes of some of these consolidations. Is that what you're saying?

Dr. DAFNY. I would like to be able to point to some successful consolidations. I co-authored a paper with a physician friend of mine, Dr. Tom Lee, called "The Good Merger," about what would be the characteristics of a good merger and I am often asked, "Can you spotlight one for us?," and I am searching still for a very nice example of it.

But I am sure that they exist.

Mr. HARPER. Would the criteria be—as we look at these and try to see whether they are positive or negative—is it better outcome for the patient? Shouldn't that be at the heart of whether it is successful or not?

Dr. DAFNY. At the heart of whether it is successful, you'd have to consider multiple dimensions. I would certainly place patient outcomes at the top of the list. But it wouldn't be the only dimension I would score it.

Mr. HARPER. Cost possibly?

Dr. DAFNY. Cost would be pretty significant, and not just the cost to the hospitals themselves but the prices that they—whether they pass through any cost savings.

Mr. HARPER. Do you believe that the consolidations will continue to increase in the future?

Dr. DAFNY. Undoubtedly.

Mr. HARPER. OK. Is there any type of healthcare consolidation that we don't know enough about to determine its impact on patients?

Dr. DAFNY. We don't know enough, in my view, about the kind of consolidation across the care continuum, if you will. In theory, if you combine hospitals and physicians and post-acute care providers and perhaps even some pharmacy elements, you might get an integrated package product that could be superior to the piecemeal approach that we have.

We don't know enough about whether that is likely to work and also whether the markets are competitive enough that the price of that product would be affordable for the value.

Mr. HARPER. Thank you very much.

At this time, the Chair will recognize the ranking member, Ms. DeGette, for 5 minutes for questions.

Ms. DEGETTE. Thank you so much, Mr. Chairman.

Dr. Dafny, I know the members of this subcommittee would love to have a copy of your paper, "The Good Merger." If you could provide that to us, that would be great.

Dr. DAFNY. With pleasure.

Ms. DEGETTE. Thanks. And then we'll help you continue to search for a good example.

As I said in my opening statement, my colleague, Tom Reed, and I have been looking into insulin prices, and I think that our investigation, the facts we've learned, have broad implications from the consolidation issues here today.

For example, the three largest PBMs control over two-thirds of the prescription drug market, and Dr. Dafny, you noted in your prepared testimony that consolidation enables PBMs to improve their bargaining position with drug companies.

But wouldn't it be fair to say that PBM consolidation also might likely result in increased prices for prescription drugs like insulin?

Dr. DAFNY. I would say that we ought to do a merger retrospective on the most recent large PBM merger and see how that affected downstream prices to consumers.

But, to the extent that a merger—that we've had more consolidation, I would expect, but I haven't seen formal statistical evidence to suggest, that prices would rise.

Ms. DEGETTE. Dr. Gaynor, I know you have got some expertise in this as well. What's your view?

Dr. GAYNOR. Well, I agree with my colleague. I think, just as you suggested, Ranking Member DeGette, there is concern. We now really only have three PBMs, in effect, in this market, and once numbers get that small it is cause for concern.

But I agree with Professor Dafny. At this point, I do not know of direct evidence on that. But it is time for a retrospective, and the Federal Trade Commission, of course, has authority through Section 6(b) of the Federal Trade Commission Act to conduct studies of this sort in the public interest. So that would certainly be a beneficial thing to pursue.

Ms. DEGETTE. That's a good avenue.

I mean, in general, if a market becomes too concentrated with one provider system, that could potentially lead to increases in prescription drug prices. Is that correct?

Dr. GAYNOR. Yes.

Ms. DEGETTE. OK. Now, these inefficiencies in the market, we think, are also affecting employer-based health insurance.

Dr. Dafny, you said the consumers in employer-based plans need to have more choices. What can we do to encourage that?

Dr. DAFNY. As you are aware, the majority of employers offer only one choice when they sponsor health insurance to their employees.

Now, larger employers who employ more than half of employees tend to offer a little bit more—two, maybe three choices. But that's not a very large set, and therefore they tend to cater to the average consumer, don't allow you to vote with your feet for the kinds of tradeoffs you want to make.

What could you do? Well, it is possible to encourage employers to offer more choices, particularly through a private exchange, which wouldn't be terribly different from what a public exchange would be.

I am not a legal expert as to the mechanisms you would use. But there's ERISA. There should be some possibility there. Many years ago, it was required to offer an HMO to employees in order to encourage that possibility, and one could imagine minor tax preferences for the variety that you offer.

Ms. DEGETTE. That's an interesting suggestion.

Dr. Gaynor, back to you. A lot of people have been talking about entirely new approaches to providing healthcare to consumers, and we are all abuzz here about this news that Amazon is making that it's entering the healthcare business.

You know, I know these ventures are still in their infancy. But do you have any thoughts about the potential of Amazon or some of these other initiatives to improve the consumer experience and bring down costs?

Dr. GAYNOR. Sure. Thank you.

Let me give one hand, other hand—a typical economist kind of response. So on the one——

Ms. DEGETTE. We'd be disappointed if you didn't.

Dr. GAYNOR. Right. Harry Truman is reported to say, "Could somebody find me a one-handed economist?"

So on the one hand—and this is the positive—a very positive aspect of this development is that executives at major corporations in the United States are paying attention to healthcare costs.

For decades, healthcare costs have been a real issue for business in the United States. But, typically, it's the domain of human resources and executives. The C–Suite hired management really have not paid a lot of attention to this.

So to have Amazon, J.P. Morgan, Berkshire Hathaway CEOs stand up and say, "This is important, we are going to do something," is very, very encouraging.

It's potentially a very innovative thing. I wish it the best of success. I hope it succeeds. We need more.

Having said that, it's not clear to me exactly what they would do. Even these companies are small relative to the overall size of the system.

There are very powerful, entrenched providers and insurers and pharma companies that can be very hard for any one employer, let alone three large employers, to deal with.

And last, again—this is the other hand here—we have seen some of this before. If you've been around long enough—and I think I have enough gray in my beard to qualify on that account—employers have stood up in public before and said, "We are going to be doing something about this," and yet here we are.

Ms. DEGETTE. Yes. OK. Thanks. Thanks, Mr. Chairman.

Mr. HARPER. Gentlewoman yields back.

The Chair will now recognize the gentleman from Texas, Mr. Barton, for 5 minutes.

Mr. BARTON. Thank you, Mr. Chairman, and thank you for holding this important hearing.

You know, there's a saying that people like myself that run for public office and have been around awhile kind of live by, and it's called "no good deed goes unpunished."

Congress keeps trying to do the right thing in healthcare. We've adopted two policies that we thought were positive, but in terms of cost they don't seem to have helped much.

One is we have a Medicare differential reimbursement between physician services provided in a physician's office and physician services provided in a hospital setting. We pay a higher rate because of the increased overhead charges if a physician works for the hospital and provides the services in the hospital.

And it appears to me that a lot of these consolidations where hospitals are purchasing physician group practices are simply to get the higher reimbursement rate. Now, that's a simplification but it sure looks that.

The other program where we've kind of been bitten in the bottom is the 340B program. We set up a system for certain hospitals that could get a discount under the 340B program. But they didn't have to pass that discount on to their patients, and we've had an explosion of hospital pharmacies applying and being accepted into the 340B program, and the oversight group that's supposedly auditing this have admitted that they don't have the personnel to really audit the program and that the cost of the program is going through the roof.

So my question is, Would it be practical and possible that, if in the case of these physician practices being purchased by hospitals, we adopted a regulation or perhaps a statute that said Medicare is going to pay the lower of the reimbursement rate before the merger, instead of they always pay higher? Would that be practical to do something like that?

Anybody can answer it.

Dr. DAFNY. I am happy to take it, Representative Barton.

You have described the extended game of whack-a-mole that Congress is playing with various healthcare sectors and probably other sectors as well, and I want to return—I will answer your question, but I want to return to the point before. If we had a competitive downstream market, you might not have to play that game as much because market forces would walk away from health plans that overpaid for the same service rendered in a hospital than in a lower-cost site of service.

So the original program was designed to cover costs, and hospitals are more costly and so you paid them more. But as you have noted, now it's being exploited.

It's my understanding that Medicare has in place the policy already for future acquisitions to not be able to bill at the hospital rate, but to bill at their initial rate or the lower rate.

The real question, I think, is about rolling back. Do you say over a certain period of time we are going to move towards site-neutral payments so as not to continue to encourage more spending in this inefficient way but recognizing that hospitals have revenue streams and employment and other things, so recognizing there may need to be some other form by which hospitals are compensated, but not in a way that distorts their incentives of where to supply services.

Mr. HARPER. OK.

Dr. GAYNOR. If I may just add something on top of what Professor Dafny said. One thing we see very commonly is that there are important spillover effects from the Medicare program onto what private health insurers do. And so a lot of private health insurers followed Medicare in adopting higher payments for hospital-based or hospital-owned practices.

So the salutary effects of reform to Medicare payment would be not just on the Medicare program itself, although, obviously, that would be hugely beneficial, but could actually have larger effects that would affect what private insurers do, because right now private insurers continue with these larger payments.

Then there are still incentives, in spite of what Medicare has done for a hospital as to acquired physician practices.

Mr. BARTON. Finally, on 340B, what if we adopted a statute or regulation that said whatever the discount is, it has to be passed through to the patient?

Dr. SCHULMAN. I think that would provide a huge incentive to go back to a practice model that we had that was much less expensive for consumers.

When 340B was passed in 1992, there were 90 safety net hospitals that were eligible. There are now over 2,000 hospitals that are eligible.

Drugs, expensive medications, in 1992 were hundreds of dollars. They are now $100,000, and so, you know, if you can make $25,000 per drug on this discount, it's just a tremendous incentive to distort the market.

Mr. BARTON. I know my time had expired. But let me ask Dr. Dafny: Baylor Scott & White merger—good or bad?

Dr. DAFNY. You know, I am under oath. But also, I don't have evidence. I do have a quote, though—a paraphrase of a quote. I was surprised to read the CEO in charge of the transaction after the fact said, "Well, once we are merged, we are going to figure out what efficiencies might be there."

In my world, I prefer you to consider that before you make a deal like this.

Mr. BARTON. Well, they're both in my district, you know, when they were separate. Now that they're merged, the biggest hospital actually in my district is the Baylor Scott & White Hospital in Waxahachie, and everybody loves them.

With that, I yield back.

Mr. HARPER. The gentleman yields back.

The Chair will now recognize the gentleman from New York, Mr. Tonko, for 5 minutes for questions.

Mr. TONKO. Thank you, Mr. Chair, and welcome to our witnesses.

I would like to start with the consolidation of providers and how that affects consumer prices.

Dr. Dafny, in your testimony you state, and I quote, "horizontal mergers of competing healthcare providers tends to raise prices." And it's not just hospitals. You note that physician market concentration has also led to higher prices.

Dr. Dafny, can you briefly explain how these different types of mergers can have harmful effects as they relate to consumer prices?

Dr. DAFNY. OK. So on a hospital side, let me start with that.

On the hospital side, hospitals have bargaining power vis-à-vis the insurers if they're unique in some way such that excluding them from an insurer network would force the insurer to have to lower premium or not be able to make sales.

If two competing hospitals that are attractive to enrollees and are substitutable for one another decide to merge, then the insurer can't play them off against each other when negotiating rates.

The insurer is likelier to need to include that joint entity in the insurer network, and therefore they can bargain for a higher price. Higher prices for healthcare services are then likely to be passed through as higher premiums.

In the case of physician practices, there are a few different factors at play. Often, that's more of a vertical transaction upstream. The hospital is acquiring the physician downstream for a variety of reasons.

One is, as Representative Barton was talking about, in order to be able to charge higher prices because the physician is now affiliated with a hospital, and that's just kind of a mechanistic element of Medicare and of other private insurance programs.

Another motivation can be to funnel more physician referrals upstream to your hospital. And then finally, to the extent that there's a horizontal element, so now you have many more, say, of a specialty group, you can do the same thing. Negotiate to have that cardiology group included in an insurance network, they can charge a higher price, and there is evidence that I cited here that there are higher commercial insurance prices as a result of hospital acquisitions of multiple physicians.

Mr. TONKO. Thank you. Thank you.

When providers merge, they often cite the potential to leverage their combined size to reduce costs. However, Dr. Dafny, you have explained that there actually isn't much evidence to support this theory in practice.

So why is that, and why are there insufficient incentives for providers to drive down costs?

Dr. DAFNY. So, I might aspire to reduce my costs following a merger. But at the same time, if I gain market power, I am going to have less of a market incentive to be efficient and be able to bring my price down. So there's less incentive to achieve it.

And then it's quite possible that there's a lack of know-how to get it done. I do cite one study by a student of mine who finds some cost reductions when a hospital system out of the area of another hospital acquires the target and can bring costs down.

However, my own research shows, using a similar sample, that they bring prices up if they acquire a hospital in the same State. So even if costs go down, those don't seem to be passed through to consumers, and most studies don't find evidence that costs do go down.

Mr. TONKO. OK. And again to Dr. Dafny, is the Medicare program particularly vulnerable to some of these problems, or do we see this in private insurance plans as well?

Dr. DAFNY. Medicare, as you know, has administered prices, so they're not as vulnerable to the post-merger price negotiations. But if you eliminate your rivals, then you also eliminate or reduce the incentive to compete on other dimensions that patients value.

So that's one point. The second point is that, of course, Medicare has its rules that we discussed that reward certain kinds of consolidation, and so they'd be vulnerable in that respect as well.

Mr. TONKO. Thank you.

And with the time that I have left, I would like to turn to consolidation amongst insurers and how they tend to raise premiums.

You did a study of what we call mega merger and found that premiums increased not just for enrollees of these insurers but even for enrollees of rival insurers.

Can you tell me how these sorts of mergers can have that ripple effect throughout the insurance market?

Dr. DAFNY. Absolutely. It's what you'd expect in any oligopolistic market where there are just a couple of competitors.

By merging, you're able to raise your price, because those customers who really like the product that you're offering can't get one from your substitute, assuming you merge with a substitute, and then that relaxes price competition for your rivals.

So it's kind of a double whammy. It is not just when hospitals merge, say in a raised price, it's not just their prices that go up. It spills over to others in the marketplace.

Mr. TONKO. Thank you very much, and with that I yield back, Mr. Chair.

Mr. HARPER. The gentleman yields back.

The Chair will now recognize the gentleman from Virginia, the vice chair of the subcommittee, Mr. Griffith, for 5 minutes.

Mr. GRIFFITH. Thank you very much, Mr. Chairman.

Dr. Gaynor, you touched on it a little bit earlier. A lot of us have concerns about having only basically three PBMs left in the market after all the mergers, and in fact in 2015 at a Judiciary Committee hearing, Professor Thomas Greene suggested it was time, just as you did, maybe for the FTC to take a look at the PBM market and the effects of consolidation. Even FDA Commissioner Scott Gottlieb has mentioned in that same hearing that he was concerned that PBMs were using their increased market power to prevent other market participants from growing or merging. So I appreciate your comments this morning.

And Mr. Chairman, I have and would ask unanimous consent to submit a letter I have received from the National Community Pharmacists Association outlining their concerns about PBM consolidation and the impact it is having on independent pharmacists.

Mr. HARPER. Without objection.

[The information appears at the conclusion of the hearing.]

Mr. GRIFFITH. Thank you, Mr. Chairman.

Is there anything you wanted to expand on that before I move to the next subject, Dr. Gaynor?

Well, thank you. I appreciate you answering those questions from Ms. DeGette. As often in some of these occasions, she and I tend to be going after the same area.

Dr. Dafny, I have a merger that has just occurred. It's a little bit unusual because the concerns primarily were, can we keep the hospital systems afloat? Two hospitals, East Tennessee and South-west Virginia, merged. We are waiting to see if costs go up. People are very concerned about it. It just happened—finalized last month. They are now Ballad Health. I would love to see your article on the good merger so I can start looking at some of those numbers.

But the concern there was one of the hospitals actually went under in one of the two systems. They're two fairly large systems, by our standards in rural America, that merged. I think they have 21 hospitals now.

So they're pretty good-sized. They're hoping they can stay afloat. That was our concern. It wasn't for financial reasons, that they were going to make more money. It's can they survive. Any comments? Do you know anything about that merger?

Dr. DAFNY. If I may, I am familiar with that transaction. In fact, I authored a public comment on it which may have been cosigned by my colleague here, Dr. Gaynor.

Mr. GRIFFITH. Were you pro or con? Dr. DAFNY. I was concerned.

Mr. GRIFFITH. OK.

Dr. DAFNY. Concerned because the hospitals sought and were granted, as you're aware, a certificate of public advantage because the Federal enforcement authorities were concerned that there was effectively mergered a monopoly in many of these areas.

And when you say the hospitals did so because they were concerned that they would remain afloat, what goes off in my head is a bell that says "price increase, price increase." How are you going to remain afloat unless you thought your cost reductions could be so substantial jointly than apart? You might be trying to use your stronger negotiating position to wrest higher prices from commercial payers, and that would make the economic environment less competitive.

I am aware the FTC did an extensive investigation, and if they had found those cost projections credible, I believe they wouldn't have tried to challenge the transaction. So I am concerned.

Mr. GRIFFITH. Yes. A number of my constituents are concerned, but we also want to make sure we have hospitals because, if you shut one down, it's not like there's another one right around the corner. It's usually around a mountain and down a mountain and up another mountain before you can get to the next hospital, and that creates concerns as well.

But I appreciate that. Dr. Gaynor, you had something? Or Dr. Schulman.

Dr. GAYNOR. If I may just add something. The use of certificates public advantage to shield merging parties from antitrust scrutiny, I think, is not the right policy. I certainly understand the vulnerabilities and the concern over communities in these kinds of situations.

But there are other ways to achieve these goals and, of course, as is well known, there is a failing firm defense for antitrust scrutiny. So that is taken into account. And the concerns that my colleague expressed certainly apply.

Mr. GRIFFITH. And I appreciate that.

Dr. Schulman, I want to blow things up. I want you to think about it because I don't have time to get an answer per se. But I want you to think about ways we can help blow up and make the market more innovative.

I really like that part of your statement and your concerns. Telemedicine—I think a big part of that is being held back by the CMS payment model and the fact it takes an act of Congress to get some new payment arrangements.

I think we have to take a look at the Stark Act. I have rural areas that are underserved, where I have room in a nursing home, but they can't set up an opportunity there for somebody from the community to come in.

I know we don't want them colluding on the nursing home patient. But we have space there that the community could use in an underserved area that we can't because we can't have telemedicine in the nursing home for a hospital an hour and a half away.

Can you give us advice—and I am out of time—but can you give us advice on what laws we need to change to make the system for reimbursement on CMS more efficient to recognizing that there are new ways to do this?

Dr. SCHULMAN. Yes, absolutely. I think we have a limited amount of time. But the idea—when I got my licensure in North Carolina, they basically explicitly told me unless I saw the patient, you know, I would be in violation of the medical practice.

So, you know, that's not the world that we live in today. We need to experiment with these kinds of innovation models, see which ones work and then deploy them.

Mr. GRIFFITH. Well, if you have language I would be very interested in it because I would like to blow up the way we do the reimbursements so we can blow up the medical system and make costs come down.

I yield back, Mr. Chairman.

Mr. HARPER. The gentleman yields back.

The Chair will now recognize the gentleman from California, Mr. Peters, for 5 minutes.

Mr. PETERS. Thank you.

Just following on Mr. Griffith's comment, in the veterans mental healthcare field, I see a huge opportunity for telemedicine, and you have got all sorts of issues with reimbursements but also with cross-State licensing, and I would certainly enjoy working with the gentleman on figuring out ways to loosen that up.

I had some questions about transparency and markets, and Mr. Gaynor, you talked about no publicly available data on total U.S. healthcare costs and utilization or prices for specific services or providers.

Do you have an idea about the first steps you'd advise Congress to take to help Federal and State authorities achieve that kind of transparency about cost and quality?

Dr. GAYNOR. Sure. Thanks for asking the question.

At present, the issue is not that the data aren't there. The data exist. We have great data from the Medicare program. CMS has done a great job with this. Medicaid resided at the State level, and private parties hold the data as well.

But on the private side, it's not easy to access, and it's not easy to access in an aggregate way. So finding a way to encourage, support, finance these activities. So one possibility, we provide financing for a national data warehouse.

Mr. PETERS. But for what? What would it look like? So——

Dr. GAYNOR. Right.

Mr. PETERS [continuing]. You know, I would want to know what the money was being spent on.

Dr. GAYNOR. Of course. Of course.

So one question is, What is actual total healthcare spending for the United States at any given point in time? Right now, we rely on estimates done very skilfully by the national health expenditure accounts at CMS. But they don't actually have comprehensive data from the private side.

So for Congress and the U.S. Government, just knowing what that is, drilling down into those data, knowing what various things cost, being able to compare Medicare, private, Medicaid, and various issues. For businesses, being able to get that information. It's surprising, but many businesses don't know what things cost, let alone individuals.

Mr. PETERS. Well, with regards to that side of it rather than the regulatory side of it, which is sort of these aggregates you describe, can we expose the markets to this information in a way that helps consumers and users make better choices?

Dr. GAYNOR. Well, sure. The saying "a little sunshine can be the best disinfectant" I think is very real, and I can give my hometown of Pittsburgh as an example. We know that we have UPMC dominating the entire market, but nobody knows actually what the prices are for anything. My colleagues, Zack Cooper and Stuart Craig and John Van Reenen, studied this issue using data from about a third of all people with private health insurance in the United States, and we found huge amounts of variation for simple things like an MRI of your knee—600 percent variation in a geographic market, but nobody knew that before.

Mr. PETERS. And Dr. Dafny, I guess you had some comments about this, too, with respect to information about ownership and financial links.

Dr. DAFNY. I do, and I have a bit of a response to your preceding question, if I may. Two acronyms—APCD and HPC. So the——

Mr. PETERS. Air Pollution Control District? Sorry. [Laughter.]

Dr. DAFNY. Probably not an exclusive acronym. Mr. PETERS. Right.

Dr. DAFNY. All Payer Claims Database and the Health Policy Commission. So my new home State of Massachusetts—I've only been there a year and a half—uses its All Payer Claims Database to create summary measures across different hospitals of average commercial prices, and not just for certain kinds of procedures but also for an entire patient life that is attributed to a given system of care. So this State has decided to take the data that it has access to and put out transparent reports on it, which enables the public to weigh in on all sorts of consolidation, both one that the dominant system partners were trying to do a couple years ago— everybody used the HPC data to make their public comments and such, the deal did not happen—and right now there's another big deal that is under consideration, and many parties are using the data that the HPC put out to try to assess that transaction.

So I think making the data available possibly through an All Payer Claims Database and possibly through State agencies who are responsible for monitoring, including notifications of material transactions, which is what the HPC does.

Mr. PETERS. So assuming that we have additional consolidation, though, any thoughts on exposing prices to consumers that can help them? Is there an example of someone doing that well?

Yes. I got four seconds.

Dr. GAYNOR. New Hampshire. Well, I agree with what Professor Dafny said about Massachusetts. They've done a great job, not just assembling the data but using it in a meaningful way and bringing it to bear.

New Hampshire also has an All Payer Claims Database, and there is some recent evidence on that by a young scholar named Zack Brown, who's joining the Economics Department at the University of Michigan, that shows that consumers actually did use the All Payer Claims Database for shopping, and it did drive prices down, and further, that providers responded to that because they knew there were some people out there looking. You don't have everybody in the market informed—just enough so that sellers know that somebody might not come to them if the price isn't competitive.

And it did have impacts, but I think we are still in the infancy of these things.

Mr. PETERS. Thank you. My time is expired. Thank you, Mr. Chairman.

Mr. HARPER. The gentleman yields back.

The Chair will now recognize the gentleman from Texas, Dr. Burgess, for 5 minutes.

Mr. BURGESS. Thank you, Mr. Chairman.

Well, as you might imagine from my opening comments, I am interested in one of the things that's kind of been left out of this discussion, is physician ownership of facilities.

And we live in a world where, unfortunately, it is possible for hospitals to own doctors but it is not possible for doctors to own hospitals, at least it hasn't been since March the 19th of 2010, when the Affordable Care Act was signed into law.

So having come from a world—my dad started a physician-owned hospital. It was in a pretty rural area of north Texas. I don't think there would have been a hospital there if he and six or seven of his partners had not decided to take the financial risk and do that. So I think there was a positive aspect to that as far as the delivery of care.

But have we really gone to the point where no longer is it reasonable, feasible, or desirable for physicians to own the facilities in which they practice?

And I will ask everyone that question. So, Dr. Gaynor, we'll start with you, and then we'll come down the line.

Dr. GAYNOR. Well, as you know, historically, physicians did own lots of hospitals, particularly smaller ones in rural areas, and that changed over a long period of time for a variety of reasons.

I don't know specific evidence on the impacts of physician ownership, in part because, as you said, it's so rare. But there is some evidence on a related area having to do with ACOs, and it seems that physician-led ACOs do tend to be more effective than in hospitalled ACOs.

So I don't want to make a great leap from there to physician ownership of all kinds of facilities, but that might suggest that there could be some gains from that.

I think we want think carefully about this, but I don't know that it's sensible to completely exclude a large group of knowledgeable participants in the healthcare system from engaging in a certain way and possibly doing some innovative and beneficial things.

Mr. BURGESS. Yes, I agree with you. It makes no sense by virtue of the academic degree that I hold, I am excluded from a certain type of business process, but lawyers and even registered nurses could engage in that practice.

Dr. Dafny, do you have anything you'd like to add?

Dr. DAFNY. I concur with Dr. Gaynor on this. I would say that I am aware of the moratorium on physician-owned specialty hospitals that would limit competition in the marketplace and so, all else equal, is likely to lead to worse service and higher prices.

That said, I would say two things. One is that I am concerned about self-referrals, not just in that context, in general. So one would want to have controls in place to try to address that.

The second is that there is research—it's not at the top of my head now—that suggests some cream skimming. You would typically want to send the cases that are riskier to a full-service hospital.

So I would just say—so I wouldn't be surprised if that were true, and that might well be really efficient. I would just say that then we ought to make sure that there are mechanisms to reimburse the hospitals appropriately.

Mr. BURGESS. I would just—and I do refer you to the article from Health Affairs from 10 years ago, because it is so well-written and so concise and puts the argument forward so reasonably—but I will just tell you, from my own experience, if I had a relatively minor case to do on a Friday morning, if I scheduled that in the hospital, I would be behind an orthopaedic procedure and possibly some other procedure and then, by golly, if I didn't start by noon or 1 o'clock, I could get bumped from an appendectomy in the emergency room, and I might spend all day waiting to get that case done.

If it's scheduled at a physician-owned outpatient center—"Doctor, we are glad to see you, your case is ready"—and literally before I've done the dictation on the first case, the next case is ready to go.

So when time is so critical, if I've got a case that reimburses at a lower rate—say, it's a self-pay or Medicaid patient—do I want to go to the facility where I am going to burn all day waiting to get it done, or do I want to go to the facility where it's going to be done quickly and then I can get onto the next?

So Dr. Schulman, I've come to you with the time I have left.

Dr. SCHULMAN. Yes. So I think at some level the generalization of this is a broader question: What's the optimal structure of the delivery system?

You know, if we go back 20 years ago, this hearing would have been about how do doctors and insurance companies work together to keep patients out of hospitals. We spent a decade working on that.

Our rhetoric has changed, and we are worried about now the tremendous costs that are coming from thinking about healthcare being centered in hospitals.

And so maybe the pendulum has really swung way too far, and the way we can save money for Medicare and everything else is by addressing utilization, paying freestanding physicians to keep patients out of hospitals, and the big challenge is now the capital that's required to do all these things with the regulatory controls, with electronic health records and everything else, is very rarely available to individual physicians.

Mr. BURGESS. And then the other thing that's left out of this discussion is the advancing complexity of what we are able to do, tools that are available today that people hadn't even thought of 20 or 25 years ago when I was in medical school. It is indeed a new world, and in some cases it's very expensive. But I, for one, am grateful some of those things are available.

Mr. Chairman, I will yield back and thank you for the recognition.

Mr. HARPER. The gentleman yields back.

The Chair will now recognize the gentlewoman from Florida, Ms. Castor, for 5 minutes.

Ms. CASTOR. Thank you, Mr. Chairman, and thank you to the witnesses who are here today.

I would like to start by addressing an implication that was left, and I just want to make sure the record is clear. We've heard an argument that the 340B program, which helps bring vital medications to the country's most vulnerable patients, has somehow caused consolidation in the healthcare industry, and since we are citing Health Affairs articles I wanted to make sure for the record we cite the 2017 Health Affairs article that found little evidence that the expansion of hospital 340B eligibility contributed to hospital acquisitions of physician practices.

Instead, researchers found that the increase in consolidation trends were tied to much broader trends, and I think that is clear and you don't have to be a healthcare expert to understand that.

But I wanted to ask you, Dr. Gaynor, considering that 340B is such a small portion of the overall healthcare sector in America, isn't it fair to say that there are larger market forces at play that are driving hospital consolidation?

Dr. GAYNOR. Thanks for the question.

Certainly, with regard to hospitals. With regard to physician practices, the effects—you're correct—are not going to be broadly across physician practices, because it doesn't touch all kinds.

But oncology in particular, there is evidence that the 340B program does lead to consolidation, and I think the issue has been not about the program itself—I think it's broadly agreed it's a beneficial and important program—but really how the payments should be structured.

Ms. CASTOR. And I think we all agree on greater transparency would be beneficial. But I just wanted to make sure that the implication was not left that 340B is the large driver of hospital consolidation. And yes, we have some issues involving oncology practices with——

Dr. GAYNOR. Yes. Yes, indeed.

Ms. CASTOR. OK.

Dr. GAYNOR. Agreed.

Ms. CASTOR. So, as we consider the trends of consolidation in healthcare overall, it is important to keep the focus on the patients and any cost savings that can be achieved and that these consolidations are not going to cost consumers more.

So my takeaway from your testimony today is there's not a lot of evidence that demonstrates that mergers are resulting in improved care and cost savings.

Dr. Dafny, you said you're still searching for examples of where consolidation has helped improve the quality of care overall, and you note that generally one of the arguments in favor of mergers is that they should enable more integrated care, which has been a goal of overall healthcare reforms, and that's rather appealing. That's an appealing argument.

What does the research say about how effective mergers have been in improving integration of care, and why?

Dr. DAFNY. Thank you for the question, Representative Castor. When it comes to looking for a good merger, I am looking for one that's good on potentially multiple dimensions. So quality would just be one of those dimensions—better quality, but a huge price increase may not be worthwhile.

You asked about whether mergers have led to more integrated care, and I will tell you that I have not seen research that has addressed that question directly, apart from when hospitals acquire physicians—and to the extent that you might think that physicians then would try to keep patients out of the hospital, and the hospital would be compensated for that somehow through the joint venture because they would be bearing some of the total risk for the span of that population—you might think spending would go down, and that is not what has happened. So to the extent that that's a measure of what the impact is of mergers on integrated care, then it's not very positive.

I will add that, if you thought that these mergers were about integrating care, you ought to see a lot more across different kinds of providers than the same old provider but in lots of different areas or next door.

Ms. CASTOR. OK.

Dr. Gaynor, could you speak a bit further to this distinction and explain why benefits integration may help or hurt consumers?

Dr. GAYNOR. Sure. Well, just to follow up on this, consolidation is not integration. The acquisition—its transactions are very involved, they're a big deal, but in some sense, that's the easy part. Once the acquisition has happened, bringing the two entities together and integrating is really hard and, unfortunately, we have just not seen that.

So why don't patients see the benefits of this? As my colleague just said, we don't tend to see more integrated care. We don't tend to see higher quality. So it just hasn't tended to be there for patients to realize, and informally one thing that market participants have said is the following:

Raising prices is easy, lowering costs is hard. And there's a lot of truth to that. Driving down costs, integrating care, improving the quality of care is actually really, really hard work. It's not easy.

Whereas, if one obtains a better negotiating position, then going around and getting a higher price is substantially easier than that.

So, unfortunately, I think that the payoffs and the incentives move in such a way that they've led market participants to take the high prices and not do the hard work.

I do want to be clear, though. This is not every transaction. I am not characterizing every transaction this way. I feel that there are good mergers out there, as well, but, again, maybe we'll find one one of these days, but I can't point to one specifically.

Ms. CASTOR. Thank you very much.

Mr. HARPER. The gentlewoman yields back.

The Chair will now recognize the gentleman from New York, Mr. Collins, for 5 minutes.

Mr. COLLINS. Thank you, Mr. Chairman. I want to thank our witnesses. I think there's a lot of agreement across the board and concern about consolidations and the like not having the impact we wanted on healthcare cost.

But back to a good merger. I have a very rural district—you know, eight counties with a declining population, thanks to our Governor. We keep losing people in New York.

So we look for a good merger. I have four, five, or six—I am going to call them a merger, I don't know, merger versus acquisition—but rural hospitals that, frankly, would have gone out of business had they not merged with a much larger healthcare system, either the city of Buffalo or city of Rochester, which reached out, took, in many cases, ownership and bought the hospital short of that hospital shutting down, and in doing so also were able to then extend orthopaedic services, cardiology services that, frankly, that small rural hospital wasn't even able to provide beforehand.

So when you say we are searching for a good merger, isn't that an example of a good merger, having a large healthcare system buy an effectively bankrupt rural hospital that was unique but, frankly, was not offering a full menu of services?

Dr. DAFNY. It might well be. I would say that only a tiny fraction of mergers generate competition concerns. Fewer than 3 percent trigger FTC investigations.

So when I say I am looking for examples, it's because case studies have yet to be published to consider all the factors. Just keeping a hospital open in and of itself is not enough, in my view, for it to be good if that was realized, again, through price increases that made healthcare less affordable for people in the region.

So I would need to do a more thorough analysis to address your question.

Mr. COLLINS. Well, I know you're from Boston and nothing—not putting it aside, if you get out to rural America, and it's a 2-hour drive—2 hours from, you know, Wyoming County or Orleans County, New York, into the city of Buffalo, and there's a single hospital and, literally, because of a decline in population, whether it's the number of births or otherwise, they don't have the ability to drive that revenue and certainly not provide, you know, the oncology, the cardiology services, to suggest you can't see a benefit when—if that hospital shuts down and those people have to drive an hour and a half to the next hospital—I am a little bit dumbfounded that you can't see the obviousness of that. And not to be insulting, unless— I mean, Boston, you can get your—other than the traffic—so I am truly concerned you can't see the obviousness of that benefit.

Dr. SCHULMAN. Yes, I think—I think we've all said, you know, each of these has to be examined on their own. North Carolina is facing a lot of the same issues. We are losing hospitals in all the rural counties, the same way in Virginia.

But at the same time, you have to look at what's happening to the behavior of the consolidating systems. We are debating right now a merger of two very large systems. The rationale was they're going to improve access to rural healthcare, but there's really actually no evidence that in fact the planning is there.

If in fact they don't do that, after the mergers there's no re-course, and we have talked about a certificate of public advantage. One of the hospitals that has operated under certificate of public advantage for a long time was Mission Hospital in Asheville, North Carolina. That certificate of public advantage is now expired, and the first thing they did was terminate their contract with the largest insurer in asking for rate increases.

So, you know, I think each of these markets has to be looked at separately. So there are advantages, and rural healthcare is a huge challenge. Some of that is because the hospitals in the city offer much higher prices—salaries to their starting docs.

Dr. DAFNY. I mean, I will add to that, if I may.

The technology of healthcare has changed. It used to be the case there wasn't much you could do for patients except for put them in the nearby hospital, quarantine them, and comfort them, and so every area had one.

But as now we've grown more specialized, it may well not be an interest of those patients to have orthopaedic advanced cardiology, oncological services at low scale. So just to say that the hospital is open and has expanded services, as I said, wouldn't be enough for me to assess whether that——

Mr. COLLINS. Well, so, again, not to belabor the point, but what they've done is, they'll send an orthopaedic one day a week to that rural hospital now that the patient's—you know, whether it's a knee or a hip—can now see a doctor 10 minutes away and not 2 hours away.

So, again, not to be confrontational, but for somebody that lives in a very rural area as I do, we can't get hung up on—you know, what's the price if there is no service? You know, talk about, you know, you can't put a price on that when there is no service.

So I think you should look more into these rural—call them mergers or acquisitions—because in my case, it's that or nothing.

So thank you very much. I yield back.

Mr. GRIFFITH [presiding]. The gentleman yields back.

I now recognize Ms. Schakowsky of Illinois for 5 minutes.

Ms. SCHAKOWSKY. Thank you. I want to apologize to our witnesses and just say I am the ranking member on another subcommittee, so I had to be there.

Let me just say, or maybe just ask, I mean, I am assuming that when we are talking about rural hospitals that those States that have expanded Medicaid, that that has been helpful in many communities that would otherwise be underserved.

Does anybody just want to say anything to that? I don't know. OK. You don't have to.

All of you have acknowledged that we've seen rapid consolidation in hospitals. Specifically, this trend has resulted in a 22 percent increase in religious hospitals between 2001 and 2016. I don't know if research has been done on this, but this is a big concern for me. As we see more and more religious hospitals merge with nonreligious hospitals, many times the nonreligious hospitals are forced to observe religious prohibitions, particularly restrictions limiting access to a full range of reproductive services by denying abortion care, birth control, fertilization treatment, and I am concerned that consolidation limits access to reproductive care, particularly for women, communities of color, and LGBT people.

Currently, one in six hospital beds are subjected to religious restrictions. Because hospitals treat the most serious health conditions like women suffering from miscarriages or ectopic pregnancies, I worry that accepting these restrictions in consolidation are causing hospitals to put business considerations before comprehensive patient care.

So my question—anyone could answer—Dr. Dafny listed it as someone, but anyone can answer—does your work touch on an increase in religious and nonreligious hospital mergers acquiring, or strategic acquisition or strategic partnerships?

Dr. DAFNY. My published research does not address that. I am aware of two findings that are relevant, and I could tell you about them.

One is there is a researcher at Kansas University, David Slusky, who has in fact shown that acquisitions of formerly nonreligious hospitals by specifically Catholic healthcare systems has led to a reduction in this slew of reproductive services that you described, would support that concern about the availability of those services.

What isn't known is whether these patients then go elsewhere to receive some of those services.

Ms. SCHAKOWSKY. If it's available in their communities. Dr. DAFNY. If it's available.

And then the second is in my own study, which is in the midst of a referee process, we have a section analysis that we did actually comparing the acquisition of hospitals by religious versus nonreligious systems, and the price increases that we find on average are not present for the acquisitions by the religious hospital systems.

Ms. SCHAKOWSKY. Yes, Dr. Gaynor.

Dr. GAYNOR. Yes, thanks. Thanks, Representative Schakowsky. That's an excellent question.

Broadly speaking, when a merger is being considered by an antitrust enforcement agency, the questions about impacts on consumers and consumer welfare and the points that you raise are certainly relevant and should be taken into account because price matters a great deal, of course, but what services are available to people and where and what the alternatives are as well as quality of care are also vitally important.

Ms. SCHAKOWSKY. I hope that will be part of the considerations when we look at the issue of consolidation because, you know, a lot of people think a hospital is a hospital and don't know that the services they may want—they may be delivering a baby, would like to have a tubal ligation at the same time, find that that is not possible and require another procedure somewhere else, if they can possibly get it.

So what effect do you think these mergers could have on access to full range of healthcare services? Do they disproportionately affect some groups more than others?

I mean, I think probably what you have said would agree that, obviously, women, but I think it's also often people of color and LGBTQ community.

As we think about ways to evaluate these mergers, then I am assuming that you all agree that other factors should be considered to ensure the full range of services that are maintained for reproductive health, and are there any red flags that would indicate the consolidation would result in reduced access to reproductive health services. I think you answered with the Kansas study. Any comments on that?

And so let me ask this, then: What steps can we take to incentivize that a full range of reproductive healthcare services are maintained?

Dr. SCHULMAN. You know, I think we talked a little bit before about the organization of care, more generally, and at some level one of your questions is, you know, why are we organizing all the care around hospitals, especially women's services, which can be done in ambulatory settings, can be done in doctors' offices?

Why did we let them get acquired by the hospital, and so how do you have a diversity of services in a community where there are different kinds of care models to address the needs of the entire population?

Ms. SCHAKOWSKY. If they're available. I mean, we are talking about overall access to these kinds of procedures which I think lots of women want, and my time is up. But I think this cannot be shoved under the table as just another thing, since women are the majority of the population.

And I yield back.

Mr. HARPER [presiding]. The gentlewoman yields back.

The Chair will now recognize the gentleman from Michigan, Mr. Walberg, for 5 minutes.

Mr. WALBERG. Thank you, Mr. Chairman, and thanks to the panel for being here.

Dr. Gaynor, on September 9th, 2011, the Ways and Means Health Subcommittee held a hearing on healthcare industry consolidation. You were a witness at that hearing.

You testified on some of these issues and on consolidation since that time. What's changed in these last 7 years? Give us some hope.

Dr. GAYNOR. I have more gray hair.

Mr. WALBERG. At least you have hair.

[Laughter.]

Dr. GAYNOR. Thank you.

Mr. WALBERG. Be gentle on the rest.

Dr. GAYNOR. So, yes. Unfortunately, I reviewed that testimony while preparing for this hearing, and I wish I had good news. But if anything, I would say that consolidation has accelerated.

One might wonder, actually, how hospitals or doctors or insurers are finding anybody left to consolidate with. Almost 30 percent of all hospitals have been involved in one or more transactions. But it's accelerated, and, like I said, I think we are finding a lot of insurance markets, hospitals, physician practice markets that are more and more concentrated, so there becomes less and less choice and less and less competition,

And 7 years ago, I think, we were hoping, again, that we'd see some of this consolidation would lead to integration, lead to some new innovative forms of organizations and delivery, and as my colleagues Dr. Schulman and Dr. Dafny have said, we just haven't seen that. There are a few instances here and there, but it just hasn't happened.

So I guess I will put the dismal in the dismal science, being an economist, and things have gotten worse, not better. I wish I could report differently.

Mr. WALBERG. At least I don't feel out of the normal, then. In my district, I can't think of a hospital that hasn't gone through some type of consolidation. All across my seven-county district and even with the medical practices, individual doctors, they're consolidating together in their own clinics, creative, until they get pulled into a hospital.

One concern that we've heard is that regulators only scrutinize consolidation when a single proposed merger is seen as large enough to attract attention based on how consolidated the market will become if it goes through. The issue, however, is that a large number of small mergers and acquisitions might not attract Government attention but eventually may limit competition in the market.

So, Dr. Gaynor, is it true that some physician acquisitions may be so small that Federal antitrust enforcers might not even know about increases in provider concentration in some markets?

Dr. GAYNOR. So thanks for the question.

Yes, that's certainly possible, because they're small enough that there's not mandatory reporting requirements under Hart-Scott-Rodino acquisition law.

But I think it's important to be aware that the agencies scrutinize these things, that they look for reports in the media, that they're actually market participants that report on things that seem troubling to them, and the number the FTC, for example, has pursued, physician consolidations—one in southeast Pennsylvania recently, another out on the West Coast—that did not meet the reporting requirements were relatively small.

There is a very tough issue about that you just identified. What happens if the initial acquisition is not that big? It doesn't look troublesome, and then the next one and the next one. But then, unfortunately, you have got a problem.

Mr. WALBERG. Especially as you think of rural areas, as my colleague mentioned.

Dr. GAYNOR. Right. Right. Again, rural areas have their own special qualities. We do want to make sure that folks that live there have access to the kind of care that they need at a reasonable price, but we do have to be concerned about untoward effects there.

So I think that looking at potential competition impacts is important. But I will be honest, that's challenging. We don't want to deny acquisitions or mergers that are potentially beneficial, and we don't want to get overly speculative.

But these things do need to be taken into account. Now, ultimately the courts—if you go to court on this—are the arbiters on this, and I think that's actually in reality a very tough standard with the courts.

Dr. SCHULMAN. In our State, North Carolina, there's two very large health systems that are trying to merge, and what's really remarkable is that no one's in charge of the private health insurance market.

You know, so we have impacts on Medicaid, impacts on Medicare, impacts on Blue Cross Blue Shield North Carolina, but there's not one office or commission like there is in Massachusetts that's responsible for monitoring the market.

So we are out trying to collect primary data to see what the impacts of these mergers might be. The idea of having an all-payer database so that you knew that this cardiology practice is the only one left in this county and is about to get acquired would be really critical information to intervene long before you get to the Federal Trade Commission.

Mr. WALBERG. Thank you. My time is expired. I yield back.

Mr. HARPER. The gentleman yields back.

The Chair will now recognize the gentlewoman from Indiana, the chair of the Ethics Committee, Mrs. Brooks, for 5 minutes.

Mrs. BROOKS. Thank you, Mr. Chairman.

I have a question, Dr. Dafny, because we started to talk a little bit about Federal enforcement, and I don't think we've talked very much about Federal enforcement.

In your written testimony, you indicate that Federal enforcement authorities have interpreted their enforcement authority in such a way that it's limited in scope. And I am a former U.S. attorney, not that I was involved in these kinds of issues, but something that caught my interest. More specifically, you indicated it's difficult to define markets in nonhorizontal transactions.

Do you think we are likely to see more nonhorizontal transactions in the healthcare market as the Department of Justice and the FTC continue to successfully challenge traditional horizontal mergers? Can you talk a bit more about the enforcement landscape?

Dr. DAFNY. Absolutely, Representative Brooks. Thanks for the question.

I have great interest in these consolidations and in the ability, or rather how limited the ability is, of antitrust enforcement to ensure competitive markets.

As you're aware, antitrust enforcers have very narrow laws to enforce, and I mentioned in my testimony and will restate here that their interpretation of Section 7, the Clayton Act, which is the statute that is used to challenge mergers, is that they must define the relevant market in which competition would be diminished by the transaction, which, if you don't dwell on it too long, sounds like a perfectly sensible thing to do, but if you're an antitrust enforcer and you're versed in all the judicial precedents, then you realize whatever market you propose in one case could affect markets you might propose in another case.

So the Federal Trade Commission has successfully won merger challenges by demonstrating that many hospital markets are quite small and a merger of rivals in a relatively narrow area, even if there are many competing providers in the general vicinity, can lead to significant price increases because people would like to be able to go to their nearest or very nearby hospital.

When you talk about nonhorizontal, now we are—suppose the different hospitals in different towns in a State seek to merge, then they arguably would not be in the same relevant antitrust market for purchase—for the patients who are going to the hospital. But an insurer facing a conglomerate that has a substantial presence throughout the State may then have to pay a higher price to that consortium of hospitals because the insurer has a broader market and wants to be sure that it can offer multisite employers a comprehensive, broad network.

So defining the relevant market when it comes to negotiating with insurers, that might be different than the market that you might use when you're thinking about patients accessing hospitals. And as a result, because of the way this has been interpreted, the Federal antitrust authorities seem very reticent to bring cases that involve combinations across different sectors, across different towns.

Mrs. BROOKS. So what type of tools do you think or knowledge might be necessary for Federal enforcement authorities to, you know, examine these proposed mergers or the mergers?

And I think you mentioned it, the public database. Or what are some tools that you think would be helpful?

Dr. DAFNY. I think trying—the bigger mountain of evidence that one can build to support that this might be problematic if in fact it is will be helpful, which is one of the reasons I called for more enforcement-focused research. When I left the Federal Trade Commission, it was the first project I started to do.

But there's not such a great volume of people who are trying to do enforcement-focused research. So I would put the data out there and allocate resources to the authorities so they can investigate this. And this is not just in hospitals, this is in pharmaceutical companies. If you merge but you're not making the same therapeutic line somehow, is competition diminished either in subsequent introductions or through the prices that you negotiate because you often negotiate with the same purchasers? There's a host of crossmarket questions that I think need to be investigated.

Mrs. BROOKS. Dr. Gaynor.

Dr. GAYNOR. Representative Brooks, very excellent question, and it's a broad issue. It's very important in healthcare. But it's important for the entire economy.

So one thing that can be done and actually needs to be done is to revise the vertical merger guidelines. If I recall, and my memory is not wonderful, I think they were last revised in 1984, and it's always been important, but particularly with so much consolidation at the horizontal level, the vertical issues, in my view, become even more prominent and salient in healthcare, but actually much more broadly as well.

So that's one very concrete thing that can be done and I think would help address this issue.

Mrs. BROOKS. Thank you.

Dr. Schulman, do you have any opinion on it?

Dr. SCHULMAN. Nothing.

Mrs. BROOKS. Thank you. I yield back.

Mr. HARPER. The gentlewoman yields back.

The Chair will now recognize the gentleman from Georgia, Mr. Carter, for 5 minutes.

Mr. CARTER. Thank you, Mr. Chairman, and thank all of you for being here. I have a great deal of respect for your academic achievements and for your expertise in this area, and I thank you for that.

There is currently a proposed merger between two companies, Luxottica—and they are an Italian company that makes eyeglass frames—and another company, Essilor, which is a French company that makes the lens itself.

So here we have a proposed merger between these two companies. They will be owning not only the eyeglass frames but also the lens, as well, and oh, by the way, they will also own EyeMed, which is the second largest vision insurer in the country, and oh, by the way, they also own retail outlets such as Pearle Vision Center, such as LensCrafters—all fine businesses, but now you have this vertical integration, if you will, of a company that owns just about everything in that area, and now they will have the ability to drive market to their different companies.

I wanted to ask you, Dr. Dafny, from a free market principle, does this make sense? I mean, is this the kind of thing we need to increase competition?

I understand that competition dictating healthcare prices or corporations that dictate prices because they control the market. Which one works better?

Dr. DAFNY. I will be the economist again and say, you know, there are two sides of this. But what you described, the vertically integrated offering, might well be much more efficient than the piecemeal offering.

So this could be beneficial. The question is, by combining, are they somehow lessening competition because might they withhold their frames from other purchasers, right?

Mr. CARTER. And that's exactly why I have a bill—imagine that—H.R. 1606, the DOC Access Bill, which addresses this, to address the free market principles and to have competition.

Full disclosure: Prior to becoming a Member of Congress, I was a practicing pharmacist for over 30 years. I have witnessed first-hand the impact that PBMs and the consolidation of PBMs and drugs stores have had on patients.

Now, this is something I—this may be the trainee training the trainer here. OK—this is the part that I think that I have seen firsthand that perhaps you haven't seen: the impact on the patient.

In my 30 years of practice of pharmacy, I was a retail pharmacist and I serviced generations of families—grandparents, parents, children, and grandchildren—and I've seen that, and they've become trustful of me and trustful of their community pharmacist, of their independent pharmacist, and you build up that relationship.

And I've had them walk into my business, when I was still practicing, literally in tears, saying, "I've got to go to another drug store. My family has used your drug store all our lives. My grandparents, my parents, they've used your pharmacies. I've used it for my children and for my grandchildren. Now I've got to go to another pharmacy because my insurance company owns that pharmacy, and they're telling me I have to go over there."

That's the real-life impact that we see through this consolidation. You mentioned before that PBMs control over 80—there are three PBMs that control over 80 percent of the market share.

Now, if you look at the mission statement of the PBMs, it will say that they are there to lower drug prices. I want to ask you, How is that working out?

If it's working out well, Dr. Schulman, why is the President identifying escalating prescription prices as being one of the things that we need to address in this country?

Dr. SCHULMAN. I think, you know, we've been talking about PBMs a little bit today. This is the least transparent business model of any of the things we've been talking about in the country.

So, in 2015, there were approximately $115 billion passed back from pharmaceutical manufacturers to PBMs and to drug distributors. Some of that was passed back to employers. Almost none of that was passed back to consumers.

Mr. CARTER. And do we know how much was passed back to employers?

Dr. SCHULMAN. We don't know.

Mr. CARTER. We don't, because—Dr. Gaynor, you said earlier that sunlight was the best transparency out there. It's infected out there. We have no transparency. Dr. Dafny, you said you were with the FTC. Why does the FTC not look into this? Why are they not doing something about this?

Dr. DAFNY. I mean, the FTC has jurisdiction to do certain things. They could do a study, and one thing we mentioned was a study of the effects of the last transaction that they did not challenge, a big merger in the——

Mr. CARTER. And this is getting worse before it gets better. Now all of a sudden we see where CVS Caremark is going to buy Aetna.

Dr. DAFNY. In fact, your description of the dental consolidation sounded very much like that integration.

Mr. CARTER. That was not intentional. But nevertheless, the point that I want to make here is that I think the one thing we may be missing is the impact it has on patients.

This does have an impact on patients. When you talk about having trust between the healthcare provider and a patient, that is invaluable. Between a doctor and a patient, that relationship is so hard to build, and yet we have insurance company—and listen, I used to call these guys crooks, and I still do when I get upset. But they're not really crooks, they're smart businesspeople. They're exploiting the system that we here in Congress are not doing our job. We are not making the changes that should be made to prevent this from happening, and it frustrates me.

Dr. SCHULMAN. Well, we've talked about the impact to patients a good bit from a lot of these consolidations. The research that we've been talking about in terms of costs and quality, most of that used claims data. Very little of that actually interviewed patients to see what happens in towns when basically they raise the parking price at the hospital to——

Mr. CARTER. And you know it does impact them. It impacts accessibility. It impacts compliance.

Dr. DAFNY. I know your time is expired, but I have to say this, which is patients are an afterthought when it comes—if they even get to be an afterthought—when it comes to discussions of consolidation. I've been privy to a number of them.

Mr. CARTER. Thank you.

Dr. GAYNOR. Just one last plug to reinforce what you said is that all these things interact in a way that makes things worse. So the issues with choice of pharmacy are compounded by lack of choice, lack of competition in health insurance.

If folks could say to the health insurance company, "Go take a hike, I will go to another insurer that's offering me access to the pharmacy," then you bet you'd get access to these pharmacies. But if the insurers don't have to compete, they won't.

Mr. CARTER. Mr. Chairman, thank you for your indulgence.

Mr. HARPER. Thank you very much. The gentleman from Georgia yields back.

The Chair will now recognize the gentleman from Pennsylvania, Mr. Costello, for 5 minutes.

Mr. COSTELLO. Thank you, Mr. Chairman.

Dr. Gaynor, during the '90s, the FTC had lost multiple hospital merger cases, but since then it appears that they have successfully challenged multiple hospital mergers after refining their approach.

Can you describe what the FTC did as a part of this retrospective study and how the FTC's approach to hospital merger review has changed?

Dr. GAYNOR. Yes. Representative Costello, thank you for the question. Good to see a fellow Pennsylvanian here, albeit——

Mr. COSTELLO. Some people would suggest that western Pennsylvania and eastern Pennsylvania, we——

Dr. GAYNOR. Yes. Yes. Albeit from that other part of the State.

Anyhow, yes. So, as you note, the FTC encountered a string of losses in the courts in which merging hospitals defended the mergers on a variety of bases, either geographic markets that were very, very broad so there were lots of potential competitors in those supposed markets that were saying, "We are not for profit, we wouldn't do anything naughty."

And the FTC, rather than prospectively going after mergers, took a break, commissioned a number of studies that looked at mergers that had actually occurred—between Evanston Northwestern Hospital and Highland Park Hospital in the suburbs of Chicago, between a number of hospitals in Wilmington, North Carolina, between Summit and Sutter in the Bay Area—and what those studies found is that those mergers which had already happened, which had been consummated and been consummated for a number of years, led to very substantial price increases. I think some of the price increases from the Bay Area merger were 40 or 50 percent or higher—Evanston Northwestern, as well.

And they didn't stop there. They looked at quality of care for patients because that's vitally important, and they did not see evidence of improvements and quality of care. Some declines, some no change. So what that did is, that gave them an evidence base to go into mergers to try and block a merger prospectively, which would change the presumption.

Now, the other thing that happened at the same time is that researchers in academia have been undertaking a lot of studies because data had become more widely available, and that added to the evidence base, as well.

And then the first merger they went after was a retrospective rather than a prospective—Evanston Northwestern and Highland Park.

So that's how they swung things around. It was a concerted effort by then-Chairman Ramirez and the staff at the FTC.

Mr. COSTELLO. Thank you.

Dr. Dafny, in your testimony you indicated you will expect that we will continue to see more consolidation. Why do you think we'll continue to see more consolidation? Will we see it more, do you predict, in standard horizontal consolidation, or will we start to see it more in vertical arrangements?

Then the final point is if you could lend any observations on the health insurance industry and how, either through acquisition of assets that then creates an insurance company or an insurance company acquiring assets by way of hospital and physician practices, what kind of dangers might be inherent in that?

Dr. DAFNY. OK. I will try to address those questions in the time remaining.

I believe we'll see more consolidation because the factors that are encouraging it don't seem to be changing. I went through some of the rewards in my testimony, but include the fact that if you merge you often have a better bargaining position, can raise your prices. You might be able to reduce your costs or think you could reduce your costs, even though there's not much evidence that that actually happens.

And there are some administrative reasons. Medicare and private insurers reward certain kinds of consolidations—say, enabling hospitals to charge more for the same service that might be supplied by a physician independently more cheaply. So I think that the factors that are driving the consolidation are still present.

I do believe that, because the Federal Trade Commission, the Department of Justice have been pretty active in horizontal merger enforcement in healthcare, that we are seeing more vertical or nonhorizontal consolidation. You're seeing hospital systems merging across different geographic areas, and their answer would be "because we think we can do that, and we think we'll be better together," and the concern is to the extent that they compete, then they might have less of an incentive to be better once they've taken out a potential entrant or a rival.

On the insurance side—now we are out of time—I would say that the results of research on insurance mergers also show premium increases when there's less competition in a market—that a hospital or a group of providers that bears risk is going to be performing a lot of the functions of an insurance company. But so long as they can't offer health plans, then they may not be able to pass all the savings along to patients.

Mr. COSTELLO. How about access to care?

Dr. DAFNY. What about access?

Mr. COSTELLO. Well, in terms—is there concern over limiting access to care on that patient?

Dr. DAFNY. Well, I think, if you eliminate essential health benefits, you would have a concern—or allow the purchase of non-qualified plans or not enforce the individual mandate—I think you may have more access issues.

Mr. COSTELLO. Thank you. I yield back. Mr. HARPER. The gentleman yields back.

That concludes our hearing. We want to say a special thank you to each of you for taking the time. It's very informative—very important topic for the future of healthcare.

And at the end of the day, we should be considering patient care and outcomes and improved cost for those patients as we look at this ahead.

I remind Members that they have 10 business days to submit questions for the record, and I ask that the witnesses agree to respond promptly should you have any questions.

With that, the hearing is adjourned.

[Whereupon, at 12:22 p.m., the committee was adjourned.]

[Material submitted for inclusion in the record follows:]

U.S. HOUSE OF REPRESENTATIVES COMMITTEE ON ENERGY AND COMMERCE

February 12, 2018

TO: Members, Subcommittee on Oversight and Investigations
FROM: Committee Majority Staff
RE: Hearing entitled "Examining the Impact of Health Care Consolidation."

I. Introduction

The Subcommittee on Oversight and Investigations will hold a hearing on Wednesday, February 14, 2018, at 10:15 a.m. in 2322 Rayburn House Office Building. The hearing is entitled "Examining the Impact of Health Care Consolidation." The purpose of this hearing is to examine consolidation trends in the health care sector, the reasons behind those trends, and the effects they have on the cost and quality of care.

II. Witnesses

- Martin Gaynor, Ph.D., E.J. Barone University Professor of Economics and Health Policy, Heinz College, Carnegie Mellon University;
- Leemore Dafny, Ph.D., Bruce V. Rauner Professor of Business Administration, Harvard Business School; and
- Kevin A, Schulman, M.D., Professor of Medicine, Gregory Mario and Jeremy Mario Professor, Duke University, Visiting Scholar, Harvard Business School.

III. Background

A. Health Care Expenditures

In 2016, U.S health care spending was estimated to be about $3.3 trillion, and the overall share of gross domestic product (GDP) related to health care spending was 17.9 percent (up from percent in 2015).[49] According to the Centers for Medicare and Medicaid Services (CMS), 32 percent of the $3.3 trillion in expenditures was spent on hospital care, 20 percent was spent on physician and clinical services, 14 percent was spent on other (including, but not limited to home health care and durable medical equipment), 10 percent was spent on prescription drugs, 8 percent was spent on government administration and net cost of health insurance, 5 percent was spent on nursing care facilities and continuing care retirement communities, 5 percent was spent on investment, and 4 percent was spent on dental services.[50] The majority—75 percent—of the $3.3 trillion in

---

[49] U.S. Dep't of Health and Human Services, Centers for Medicare & Medicaid Services, *National Health Expenditures 2016 Highlights* (Dec. 2017), *available at* https://www.cms.gov/Research-Statistics-Data-and-Systems/Statistics-Trends-and-Reports/NationalHealthExpendData/Downloads/highlights.pdf.

[50] U.S. Dep't of Health and Human Services, Centers for Medicare & Medicaid Services, *The Nation's Health Dollar ($3.3 Trillion), Calendar Year 2016: Where it Came From, Where it Went* (Dec. 2017), *available at* https://www.cms.gov/Research-Statistics-Data-and -Systems/Statistics-Trends-and-Reports/NationalHealthExpendData/Downloads/PieChartSourcesExpenditures.pdf.

expenditures was paid for by health insurance (34 percent by private health insurance, 20 percent by Medicare, 17 percent by Medicaid, and 4 percent by the U.S. Department of Veterans Affairs (VA), the U.S. Department of Defense (DOD), and the Children's Health Insurance Program (CHIP)).[51]

According to a Kaiser Family Foundation analysis of National Health Expenditure data released by CMS, total health expenditures have increased substantially over the past several decades.[52] Indeed, data released by CMS indicates that total health expenditures in the U.S. were about $721 billion in 1990, $1.4 trillion in 2000, $2.4 trillion in 2008, and $3.3 trillion in 2016.[53] Moreover, on a per capita basis, health spending has also grown—increasing from $8,412 in 2010 to $10,348 in 2016.[54] Although health care expenditures have continued to increase at a rapid pace, U.S. health care spending increased in 2016 at a slower rate than in previous years (in 2016, spending on health care increased by 4.3 percent compared to 5.1 percent in 2014 and 5.8 percent in 2015).[55]

Many different factors influence health care spending, including, but not limited to, population aging, prices, policy changes, and public and private initiatives.[56] In June 2017, the Medicare Payment Advisory Commission (MedPAC) reported that certain types of consolidation in the health care industry may contribute to higher commercial prices for health care and results in increased health care costs for Medicare and commercial

---

[51] *Id.*
[52] Rabah Kamal and Cynthia Cox, Peterson-Kaiser Health System Tracker, *How has U.S. spending on health care changed over time?* (Dec. 20, 2017), *available at* https://www.healt hsystemtracker.org/chart-collection/u-s-spending-healthcare-changed-time/#item-total-healt h-expenditures-increased-substantially-past-several-decades_2017.
[53] *Id.*
[54] *Id.*
[55] Micah Hartman, et al., *National Health Care Spending in 2016: Spending and Enrollment Growth Slow After Initial Coverage Expansions*, HEALTH AFFAIRS, Vol. 37, No. 1 (Dec. 6, 2017), *available at* https://www.healthaffairs.org/doi/full/10.1377/hlthaff.2017.1299.
[56] Aaron C. Catlin and Cathy A. Cowan, *History of Health Spending in the United States, 1960-2013* (Nov. 19, 2015), *available at* https://www.cms.gov/Research-Statistics-Data-and-Systems/Statistics-Trends-and-Reports/NationalHealthExpendData/Downloads/HistoricalNHEPaper.pdf; Sean P. Keehan, et al., *National Health Expenditure Projections, 2016-25: Price Increases, Aging Push Sector to 20 Percent of Economy*, HEALTH AFFAIRS (Mar. 2017), *available at* https://www.ssc.wisc.edu/~gwallace/Papers/Health%20Aff-2017-Keehan-hlthaff.2016.1627 %20(1).pdf.

insurers.[57] MedPAC noted that "[m]arkets with greater physician-practice consolidation have had greater increases in physician prices" and "[c]ommercial insurers also pay higher rates to hospitals with greater market power."[58] The Commission has expressed concerns that the market concentration effects of provider consolidation may lead to increased Medicare spending if commercial prices are "imported" into the program.[59]

B. Health Care Consolidation

i. Overview

There has been consolidation in the health care industry for decades.[60] Consolidation can occur in a variety of different ways, including horizontal and vertical mergers of hospitals, physicians, health insurers, pharmaceutical companies, pharmaceutical benefit managers, pharmacies, and other stakeholders. While there can be efficiencies from consolidation, including reducing duplicative services and improving the quality of care, consolidation also can increase the market power of certain firms and result in increased prices or reduced quality of care.[61] Some experts have raised concerns about increased consolidation in certain parts of the health care industry and its impact on competition. For example, in May 2016, the former Chairwoman of the Federal Trade Commission (FTC), Edith

---

[57] Medicare Payment Advisory Commission (MedPAC), *Report to the Congress: Medicare and the Health Care Delivery System, Chapter 10: Provider Consolidation: The Role of Medicare Policy* (June 2017).

[58] Medicare Payment Advisory Commission (MedPAC) Staff, *Why Have Medicare Costs Grown So Much Slower Than the Costs of Employer-Sponsored Insurance?* (Sept. 11, 2017), available at http://medpac.gov/-blog-/why-have-medicare-costs-grown-so-much-slower-than-the-cost-of-employer-sponsored-insurance/2017/09/11/why-have-medicare-costs-grown-so-much-slower-than-the-cost-of-employer-sponsored-insurance.

[59] *Id.*

[60] Medicare Payment Advisory Commission (MedPAC), *Report to the Congress: Medicare and the Health Care Delivery System, Chapter 10: Provider Consolidation: The Role of Medicare Policy*, at 295 (June 2017).

[61] American Hospital Association, *Hospital Mergers: Foundation for a Modern, Efficient and High-Performing Health Care System of the Future* (Jan. 2017); Martin Gaynor, E.J. Barone Professor of Economics and Health Policy, Heinz College, Carnegie Mellon University, *Statement before the Committee on Ways and Means Health Subcommittee, U.S. House of Representatives* (Sept. 9, 2011), available at https://waysandmeans.house.gov/UploadedFiles/Gaynor_Testimony_9-9-11_Final.pdf.

Ramirez, expressed concerns about the "rapid rate of consolidation among healthcare providers."[62] Moreover, in October 2017, the Trump Administration issued an Executive Order to foster greater competition in the health care markets and directing the Administration to "continue to focus on promoting competition in healthcare markets and limiting excessive consolidation throughout the healthcare system."[63]

Many segments of the health care market are highly concentrated—one researcher found that, in 2016, 90 percent of Metropolitan Statistical Areas were highly concentrated for hospitals, 65 percent for specialist physicians, 39 percent for primary care physicians, and 57 percent for insurers.[64] According to Kaufman Hall, there were 115 transactions involving hospitals and health systems in 2017—a thirteen percent increase since 2016 and the highest amount in recent history.[65] Although the number of transactions in 2017 involving hospitals and health systems was similar to the number of transactions in 2015, the aggregated revenue of the transacted organizations was almost double.

Deals among hospitals and health systems[66]

Year	Transacted Revenue ($ billions)	Number of Transactions
2017	$63,186	115
2016	$31,288	102
2015	$32,028	112
2014	$23,098	102
2013	$31,328	98

---

[62] Federal Trade Commission, *Keynote Address of FTC Chairwoman Edith Ramirez, Antitrust in Healthcare Conference* (May 12, 2016), *available at* https://www.ftc.gov/system/files/documents/public_statements/950143/160519antitrusthealthcarekeynote.pdf.
[63] Exec. Order 13813, 82 Fed. Reg. 48385 (Oct. 17, 2017), *available at* https://www.gpo.gov/fdsys/pkg/FR-2017-10-17/pdf/2017-22677.pdf.
[64] Brent D. Fulton, *Health Care Market Concentration Trends in the United States: Evidence and Policy Responses*, HEALTH AFFAIRS, Vol. 36, No. 9 (Sept. 2017).
[65] Kaufman Hall, *2017 in Review: The Year M&A Shook the Healthcare Landscape* (2018), *available at* https://www.kaufmanhall.com/sites/default/files/2017-in-Review_The-Year-that-Shook-Healthcare.pdf.
[66] *Id.*

In addition to hospital and health system mergers, there has been consolidation in other parts of the health care industry as well. Physician groups, health insurers, pharmaceutical companies, pharmaceutical benefit managers (PBMs), pharmacy services, and other stakeholders have engaged in vertical and horizontal integration.[67] Following mergers within the PBM industry over the past decade, the largest three PBMs accounted for more than 70 percent of market revenues in 2016.[68] Over the past few years, there have been many mergers and acquisitions in the pharmaceutical industry too. According to an April 2017 report by IBIS World, the four largest brand name pharmaceutical manufacturers accounted for over 40 percent of total industry revenue.[69] Similarly, according to a March 2017 report by IBIS World, the top three generic pharmaceutical manufacturing companies in the United States accounted for 21.6 percent of industry revenue in 2017.[70]

To provide a brief overview of some of types of consolidation in the hospital, physician, and insurance markets, the next two sections of this memorandum discuss three examples of horizontal and vertical integration, including: (1) horizontal hospital integration; (2) vertical hospital-physician integration; and (3) horizontal insurer integration. This list is not provided as an exhaustive list of the different types of consolidation occurring in the health care industry.

---

[67] See e.g., Federal Trade Commission, Health Care Division, Bureau of Competition, *Overview of FTC Actions in Health Care Services and Products* (Sept. 2017); Federal Trade Commission, Health Care Division, Bureau of Competition, *Overview of FTC Actions in Pharmaceutical Products and Distribution* (Sept. 2017).

[68] Evan Hoffman, *IBISWorld Industry Report OD4620: Pharmacy Benefit Management in the US*, IBISWORLD (Nov. 2016).

[69] Kelsey Oliver, *IBISWorld Industry Report 32541a: Brand Name Pharmaceutical Manufacturing in the US*, IBISWORLD (April 2017).

[70] Kelsey Oliver, *IBISWorld Industry Report 32541b: Generic Pharmaceutical Manufacturing in the US*, IBISWORLD (Mar. 2017); *See also* Marc-Andre Gagnon and Karen D. Volesky, *Merger mania: mergers and acquisitions in the generic drug sector from 1995 to 2016, Globalization and Health* (2017), available at https://www.ncbi.nlm.nih.gov/pmc/articles/PMC5567637/pdf/12992_2017_Article_285.pdf.

ii. Hospital and Hospital-Physician Consolidation

Hospitals and providers have been merging for decades.[71] According to Irving Levin Associates, Inc., there were 1,412 hospital deals involving 3,009 total hospitals from 1998 to 2015.[72] Although the number of announced hospital mergers and acquisitions stayed relatively consistent between 2002 and 2009 with fewer than 60 transactions a year, the number of announced hospital mergers per year began to increase following the Affordable Care Act.[73]

Over the past ten years, hospitals have also acquired a significant number of physician practices. According to a 2015 report by the Government Accountability Office (GAO), the number of vertically consolidated hospitals increased from about 1,400 in 2007 to 1,700 in 2014, and the number of vertically consolidated physicians nearly doubled during that same period from about 96,000 to 182,000.[74] Similarly, from 2007 to 2013, Medicare spending in hospital outpatient departments (HOPDs) increased, rising at an annual rate of 8.3 percent—substantially faster than the 5.8 percent growth rate in total Medicare Part B spending.[75] In November 2017, an analysis by Avalere Health showed that the number of physicians employed by hospitals increased by 49 percent between 2012 and 2015.[76]

---

[71] Federal Trade Commission, *"Hospital Consolidation: The Good, The Bad, and The Ugly,"* Keynote Address by Maureen K. Ohlhausen, Commissioner, Federal Trade Commission (Mar. 13, 2013), available at https://www.ftc.gov/system/files/documents/public_statements/115852/130313hospitalconsolidationspeech.pdf.

[72] American Hospital Association, *Trendwatch Chartbook 2016 Organizational Trends, Chart 2.9: Announced Hospital Mergers and Acquisitions, 1998-2015* (2016), available at https://www.aha.org/system/files/research/reports/tw/chartbook/2016/chart2-9.pdf.

[73] *Id.*; *See also* Matt Schmitt, *Do Hospital Mergers Reduce Costs?*, UCLA ANDERSON (Jan. 16, 2017), available at https://pdfs.semanticscholar.org/0005/6b7e6d5e18a0fa38e07472 65e86b277ff368.pdf.

[74] U.S. Gov't Accountability Office, *Medicare: Increasing Hospital-Physician Consolidation Highlights Need for Payment Reform*, GAO-16-189 (Dec. 2015).

[75] *Id.* at 1.

[76] Physician Advocacy Institute, *Implications of Hospital Employment of Physicians on Medicare & Beneficiaries, Analysis by Avalere Health, LLC* (Nov. 2017), available at http://www.physiciansadvocacyinstitute.org/Portals/0/assets/docs/PAI_Medicare%20Cost% 20Analysis%20--%20FINAL%2011_9_17.pdf.

Announced Hospital Mergers and Acquisitions, 1998-2015[77]

Year	Number of Deals
1998	139
1999	110
2000	86
2001	83
2002	58
2003	38
2004	59
2005	51
2006	57
2007	58
2008	60
2009	52
2010	72
2011	93
2012	107
2013	88
2014	99
2015	102

Hospitals and providers have many arguments justifying consolidation, including improved coordination, enhanced efficiencies, reduced costs of capital, economies of scale, elimination of duplicative services, reduced regulatory burdens and practice management responsibilities for physicians, reduced regulatory costs, expanded scope of services available to patients, and improved quality of care.[78] At the same time, some research shows that consolidation of certain providers and hospitals may increase the cost of care and does not necessarily improve quality.

---

[77] American Hospital Association, *Trendwatch Chartbook 2016 Organizational Trends, Chart 2.9: Announced Hospital Mergers and Acquisitions, 1998-2015* (2016); *See also* Leemore Dafny, Ph.D., *Hospital Industry Consolidation – Still More to Come?*, NEW ENGLAND JOURNAL OF MEDICINE (Jan. 16, 2014).

[78] Medicare Payment Advisory Commission (MedPAC), *Report to the Congress: Medicare and the Health Care Delivery System, Chapter 10: Provider Consolidation: The Role of Medicare Policy*, at 290 (June 2017); American Hospital Association, *Hospital Mergers: Foundation for a Modern, Efficient and High-Performing Health Care System of the Future* (Jan. 2017).

- In June 2017, MedPAC reported that hospital markets are highly consolidated. MedPAC wrote,

> The literature generally finds that horizontal hospital consolidation leads to higher inpatient prices. Gaynor and colleagues summarize the findings: 'Mergers between rival hospitals are likely to raise the price of inpatient care and these effects are larger in concentrated markets. The estimated magnitudes are heterogenous and differ across market settings, hospitals, and insurers' (Gaynor et al. 2014).[79]

On the impact of vertical physician-hospital consolidation on price, MedPAC stated that:

> Vertical physician-hospital consolidation increases both commercial and Medicare prices paid for physician services. Commercial physician prices can increase because of the market power of the hospitals owning the practices. Medicare prices increase as the program pays a physician fee and a hospital facility fee for an office visit that would have been paid only a physician fee if the visit had been provided in a freestanding physician office.[80]

With respect to provider consolidation, MedPAC indicated that,

> [T]he literature fails to find strong evidence that financial consolidation consistently leads to lower costs or higher quality (Burns et al. 2013, Gaynor and Town 2012b, Gaynor et al. 2017). While some integrated entities report strong cost or quality performance, in other cases, systems may financially integrate for the tangible financial benefits of market power and Medicare facility fees rather than a cultural commitment to affordable integrated care.[81]

---

[79] Medicare Payment Advisory Commission (MedPAC), *Report to the Congress: Medicare and the Health Care Delivery System, Chapter 10: Provider Consolidation: The Role of Medicare Policy*, at 299 (June 2017).
[80] *Id.*
[81] *Id.* at 290.

- In 2018, research from the Kellogg School of Management at Northwestern University found that "from 2007 to 2013, almost 10 percent of physician practices in the [insurance-company data that they acquired for the study] were acquired by a hospital. Once acquired, prices for the services provided by those physicians rose an average of 14 percent."[82] The researchers also found that the "way the laws are currently written and enforced, the antitrust agency is unlikely *to even know* about the increases in provider concentration."[83]
- In 2016, Milliman examined the cost of cancer care and found that one "trend contributing to the increase in cancer care costs has been the shift in the site of chemotherapy infusion deliver from generally lower-cost physician office settings to generally higher-cost hospital outpatient settings."[84]

Federal and state policies can impact a hospital and a physician group's decision regarding whether to vertically integrate by providing financial, or other, incentives to consolidate.[85] For example, historically, the Medicare program's Hospital Outpatient Prospective Payment System (HOPPS) paid more for the same services provided at hospital outpatient departments than in other settings, such as a physician office or ambulatory

---

[82] Cory Capps, David Dranove, and Christopher Ody, *When Healthcare Providers Consolidate, Medical Bills Rise*, Kellogg Insight (Feb. 1, 2018), *available at* https://insight.kellogg.northwestern.edu/article/when-healthcare-providers-consolidate-medical-bills-rise.
[83] *Id.*
[84] Kathryn Fitch, RN, Med, Pamela M. Pelizzari, MPH, and Bruce Pyenson, FSA, MAAA, *Cost Drivers of Cancer Care: A Retrospective Analysis of Medicare and Commercially Insured Population Claim Data 2004-2014*, Commissioned by the Community Oncology Alliance, MILLIMAN (Apr. 2016), *available at* http://www.siteneutral.org/wp-content/uploads/2016/06/1_COA-Study.-Cost-Drivers-of-Cancer-Care.pdf.
[85] *See, e.g.*, Martin Gaynor, H. John Heinz III College, Carnegie Mellon University, Farzad Mostashari, Aledade, Inc., Paul Ginsburg, The Brookings Institution, University of Southern California, *Making Health Care Markets Work: Competition Policy for Health Care, Actionable Policy Proposals for the Executive Branch, Congress, and the States* (April 2017), *available at* https://www.brookings.edu/research/making-health-care-markets-work-competition-policy-for-health-care/.

surgery center.[86] Some experts argued that the payment differential accelerated consolidation of providers, while other stakeholders questioned the concerns about consolidation.[87] In 2015, GAO examined Medicare payment policies and concluded that "regardless of what has driven hospitals and physicians to vertically consolidate, paying substantially more for the same services when performed in an HOPD rather than a physician office provides an incentive to shift services that were once performed in physician offices to HOPDs after consolidation has occurred."[88] In 2015, Congress enacted the Bipartisan Budget Act and moved toward partially equalizing rates between new off campus hospital outpatient departments and physician practices.[89] MedPAC continues to recommend that Congress establish site-neutral payments for all sites of care to protect the Medicare program from the cost of physician-hospital consolidation.[90]

Another federal policy that may create incentives for certain types of hospital-physician consolidation is the 340B Drug Pricing Program (340B program).[91] For example, a 2018 article published in the New England Journal of Medicine found that: "[t]he 340B Program has been associated with hospital-physician consolidation in hematology-oncology and with more hospital-based administration of parenteral drugs in hematology-oncology and ophthalmology."[92] Similarly, a 2017 report issued by the

---

[86] *See* Letter from Fred Upton, Chairman, H. Committee on Energy and Commerce, and Joseph R. Pitts, Chairman, Subcommittee on Health, H. Committee on Energy and Commerce, to Member of the Health Care Community, 114th Congress (Feb. 5, 2015).

[87] *Id.*

[88] U.S. Gov't Accountability Office, *Medicare: Increasing Hospital-Physician Consolidation Highlights Need for Payment Reform*, GAO-16-189 (Dec. 2015).

[89] Medicare Payment Advisory Commission (MedPAC), *Report to the Congress: Medicare and the Health Care Delivery System, Chapter 10: Provider Consolidation: The Role of Medicare Policy*, at 305 (June 2017).

[90] *Id.* at 292 & 305.

[91] *See, e.g.*, Martin Gaynor, H. John Heinz III College, Carnegie Mellon University, Farzad Mostashari, Aledade, Inc., Paul Ginsburg, The Brookings Institution, University of Southern California, *Making Health Care Markets Work: Competition Policy for Health Care, Actionable Policy Proposals for the Executive Branch, Congress, and the States*, at 12 (April 2017).

[92] Sunita Desai, Ph.D and J. Michael McWilliams, M.D., Ph.D, *Consequences of the 340B Drug Pricing Program*, THE NEW ENGLAND JOURNAL OF MEDICINE (Feb. 9, 2018).

National Academies Press described how the 340B program may act to encourage consolidation of health care providers:

> For example, hospital-affiliated outpatient practices that qualify for 340B discounts can purchase drugs at reduced costs while still receiving full reimbursement for them in addition to their ability to charge facility fees. Conversely, community oncology practices that do not qualify for 340B discounts operate on lower per person-per treatment margins derived from the administration of the drugs they purchase, including the revenue generated off buy and bill reimbursements and the ability to charge facility fees (Polite et al., 2014). These disparities in revenue-generating incentives may act to encourage the consolidation of health care providers (baker et al., 2014; Cutler and Scott-Morgan, 2013). For example, there has been significant growth in 340B eligibility among outpatient clinics affiliated with 340B participating hospitals preceding and following [the Patient Protection and Affordable Care Act] implantation. As a result, GAO estimates that 340B discounts apply to 50 percent of cancer drugs sold and paid for by Medicare part B (GAO, 2015).[93]

iii. Insurer Consolidation

The landscape of competition in the health insurance industry has changed over the years and there has been a significant amount of consolidation in the market—the estimated national market share of the largest four insurers increased from 74 percent in 2006 to 83 percent in 2014.[94] Because health insurance generally operates within different regions, competition in the health insurance market is best examined by

---

[93] National Academies Press, *Making Medicines Affordable: A National Imperative*, Pre-publication Copy at 113 (Nov. 2017).

[94] Leemore Dafny, Ph.D, Professor of Strategy, Herman Smith Research Professor of Hospital and Health Services, Director of Health Enterprise Management, Kellogg School of Management, Northwestern University, Before the Senate Committee on the Judiciary, Subcommittee on Antitrust, Competition Policy, and Consumer Rights on *"Health Insurance Industry Consolidation: What Do We Know From the Past, Is it Relevant in Light of the ACA, and What Should We Ask?"* (Sept. 22, 2015), *available at* https://www.judiciary.senate.gov/imo/media/doc/09-22-15%20Dafny%20Testimony%20Updated.pdf.

analyzing local market concentration.[95] According to a study released by the American Medical Association, in 2016, 43 percent of Metropolitan Statistical Areas had at least one insurer with at least a 50 percent share of the market.[96] Similarly, according to the Kaiser Family Foundation, enrollment in Medicare Advantage is highly concentrated in a limited number of companies in both national and local markets.[97] For example, in 2015, four insurers controlled 61 percent of the Medicare Advantage market nationally.[98] Likewise, in 2014, Avalere Health found that there was significant consolidation in the number of Medicare Part D standalone prescription drug plans (PDPs) and that offerings would decrease by approximately 14 percent in 2015 due to consolidation of offerings by the main plan sponsors—from 1,169 PDPs in 2014 to 1,001 PDPs in 2015.[99] In 2017, MedPAC reported that "[i]n 2017, plan sponsors are offering 746 PDPs, a 16 percent decrease from 2016, and 1,734 [Medicare Advantage Prescription Drug Plans (MA-PDs)], a 3 percent increase from 2016. PDP reductions reflect mergers and acquisitions among plan sponsors as well as consolidation of plan offerings into fewer, more widely differentiated

---

[95] Martin Gaynor, H. John Heinz III College, Carnegie Mellon University, Farzad Mostashari, Aledade, Inc., Paul Ginsburg, The Brookings Institution, University of Southern California, *Making Health Care Markets Work: Competition Policy for Health Care, Actionable Policy Proposals for the Executive Branch, Congress, and the States*, at 12 (April 2017).

[96] Andis Robeznieks, *Health insurance markets are highly concentrated, new report reveals*, AMERICAN MEDICAL ASSOCIATION NEWS (Oct. 23, 2017), *available at* https://wire.ama-assn.org/ama-news/health-insurance-markets-are-highly-concentrated-new-report-reveals.

[97] Gretchen Jacobson, Anthony Damico, Tricia Neuman, *Medicare Advantage 2017 Spotlight: Enrollment Market Update* (Jun. 6, 2017), *available at* https://www.kff.org/medicare/issue-brief/medicare-advantage-2017-spotlight-enrollment-market-update/.

[98] Leemore Dafny, Ph.D, Professor of Strategy, Herman Smith Research Professor of Hospital and Health Services, Director of Health Enterprise Management, Kellogg School of Management, Northwestern University, Before the Senate Committee on the Judiciary, Subcommittee on Antitrust, Competition Policy, and Consumer Rights on *"Health Insurance Industry Consolidation: What Do We Know From the Past, Is it Relevant in Light of the ACA, and What Should We Ask?"* (Sept. 22, 2015), *available at* https://www.judiciary.senate.gov/imo/media/doc/09-22-15%20Dafny%20Testimony%20 Updated.pdf.

[99] Kelly Brantley, *Avalere Analysis Reveals Significant Consolidation Amoung PDPs*, AVALERE (Sept. 22, 2014), *available at* http://avalere.com/expertise/managed-care/insights/avalere-analysis-reveals-significant-consolidation-among-pdps/.

products."[100] MedPAC also reported, however, that beneficiaries continue to have broad choice among plans.[101]

C. Federal Trade Commission and Department of Justice

Antitrust authorities, including the FTC and the Department of Justice (DOJ), are best positioned to investigate and challenge horizontal mergers of providers that supply similar services in geographic proximity.[102] The FTC was initially unsuccessful in challenging provider mergers in the 1990s.[103] As a result, FTC utilized economists to review past hospital mergers after federal courts relied on broad geographic markets to thwart FTC and DOJ merger challenges.[104]

The FTC now focuses on "whether a merger is likely to affect the ability of an *insurer*— the company directly paying for the services—to avoid a price increase by excluding the hospitals in a given geographic area from its network of providers."[105] For example, since 2013, there have been multiple appellate court decisions "validating the [FTC's] approach to analyzing virtually every aspect of provider combinations, from market definition to competitive effects, failing firms, and efficiencies."[106]

Recently, the DOJ successfully blocked merger deals between Anthem Inc. and Cigna Corporation and between Aetna Inc. and Humana Inc.[107] According to DOJ's press release regarding the Anthem-Cigna merger, the merger would have "stifled competition, harming consumers by increasing health insurance prices and slowing innovation aimed at lower the costs of

---

[100] Medicare Payment Advisory Commission (MedPAC), *Report to Congress: Medicare Payment Policy, Chapter 14: Status report on the Medicare prescription drug program (Part D)* (Mar. 2017).
[101] *Id.*
[102] *See* Deborah L. Feinstein, Director, Bureau of Competition, FTC, *Remarks at AAI Healthcare Roundtable* (Feb. 22, 2017), *available at* https://www.ftc.gov/system/files/documents/public _statements/1120623/feinstein_aai_speech_2-22-17.pdf.
[103] *Id.*
[104] *Id.*
[105] *Id.*
[106] *Id.*
[107] A.M. Best Company, *Best's Briefing, Market Segment Outlook: U.S. Health* (Jan. 2, 2018).

healthcare."[108] Similarly, according to DOJ's press release regarding the Aetna-Humana merger, the merger would have "stifled competition and led to higher prices and lower quality health insurance."[109] Because DOJ's actions blocking these mergers seems to have halted large-scale mergers of health insurers, some analysts have speculated that the new focus will likely be on vertical integration—"a merging of health care functions among providers, payers, care management, and finance."[110]

iv. Issues

The following issues may be examined at the hearing:

- Why is consolidation occurring in the health care market?
- What sectors of the health care market has seen the most amount of consolidation?
- What is the impact of consolidation on patients and innovation?
- Are there any federal laws or policies that incentive consolidation in the health care market?

v. Staff Contacts

If you have any questions regarding the hearing, please contact Natalie Turner, Lamar Echols, or Jen Barblan of the Committee staff at (202) 225-2927.

---

[108] U.S. Dep't of Justice, Office of Public Affairs, *U.S. District Court Blocks Anthem's Acquisition of Cigna* (Feb. 8, 2017), *available at* https://www.justice.gov/opa/pr/us-district-court-blocks-anthem-s-acquisition-cigna.

[109] U.S. Dep't of Justice, Office of Public Affairs, U.*S. District Court Blocks Aetna's Acquisition of Humana* (Jan. 23, 2017), *available at* https://www.justice.gov/opa/pr/us-district-court-blocks-aetna-s-acquisition-humana.

[110] A.M. Best Company, *Best's Briefing, Market Segment Outlook: U.S. Health* (Jan. 2, 2018).

HEALTH AFFAIRS BLOG: BUILDING SOMETHING WORTH BUILDING FOR ALL PATIENTS

Michael Burgess

MARCH 24, 2008
10.1377/hblog20080324.000367

Editor's Note

Today, Rep. Michael Burgess (R-TX) kicks off a series of posts on Jon Gabel's article "Where Do I Send Thee? Does Physician-Ownership Affect Referral Patterns To Ambulatory Surgical Centers?," published March 18 on the Health Affairs Web site. *The series will also feature posts from Jerry Cromwell and Chris Cassel.* To paraphrase the great American architect, Frank Lloyd Wright: no man should write about building who has not himself built something worth building. As a physician who helped build an ambulatory surgery center (ASC), I conform to Mr. Wright's formula and am glad to pen some thoughts about my personal experiences with the facility. Let me begin by stipulating that I am neither a statistician, an economist, nor an academic. I have, however, practiced twenty-five years' worth of medicine. My experience is far-ranging: from a multispecialty practice, to a solo practice, and then in a single-specialty group. It was as a part of this single-specialty group I helped organize and start an ASC in my Texas hometown. And now, by virtue of the fact that I have been elected to Congress, one could argue that I've become an expert in almost anything. Therefore, I am grateful to have the opportunity to provide some alternative insights into the conclusions outlined in the piece by Jon Gabel and colleagues titled "Where Do I Send Thee? Does Physician-Ownership Affect Referral Patterns to Ambulatory Surgery Centers?" While the overall piece is thoughtful, I take issue with some of the conclusions. First and foremost, it is unfair to assume that self-pay patients fall into one of two categories: those seeking cosmetic surgery or those who are wealthy. There are also those who lack health insurance. Like other patients, the uninsured require and request surgery as well. In my own practice of obstetrics and gynecology, it was in dealing with patients who lacked health insurance where the payment disparity among different facilities became most apparent. Many times I encountered patients who desired operations, such as tubal ligation, but lacked health insurance. If they chose to pay for this operation, our local hospital would ask them to pay up front between $8,000 and $12,000. If, however, they were to make the same inquiry at an outpatient surgical center, they would find the total facility fee to be in the range of $1,000. My own modest fee for this procedure was in the neighborhood of $400, which would be unchanged whether the surgery was performed in a hospital facility or an ASC. In response to these facts, I would simply ask the rhetorical question: in which scenario was I more likely to be paid my fee? That in which the patient had paid $1,000 for the facility or a figure about ten times as high? Invariably the patient's finances would be depleted by the hospital charge, and the physician's fee would often go unpaid. Thus, if a patient with no insurance presented to my practice for an elective procedure, my likelihood of receiving compensation might, in fact, be increased if the patient were referred to an ASC, regardless of ownership.

Ownership Encourages Quality

Payment disparities are certainly a challenge. But, there are many other health care concerns today, including the issues of quality of care and payment for performance. One of the most controversial and complex subjects is physician-ownership of medical facilities, as evidenced by Gabel and colleagues' discussion. There is an old axiom that says no one ever checks the water in the battery of a rental car. There is a lot to be said for pride of ownership in any facility, including one's own office or one's ASC.

The Relative Efficiency of ASCs

Paperwork and policy are also problems when it comes to modern-day health care. In my own twenty-five years of clinical practice, I had multiple struggles with hospital administration. Indeed, sometimes the conventional wisdom was that my local hospital behaved like an absentee landlord. I recall very vividly a five-year effort to get filtered drinking water for my hospitalized patients. It is not a battle I would like to relive at any point in the future. Additionally, timing and schedules are critical parts of any medical practice. I was fortunate to have a robust roster of patients. So I began scheduling minor procedures on a day that I typically took out of the office. If I were to do four procedures at my local hospital, turnover time after each case would approach one hour. As a consequence, I could complete those four extra cases each week, but it would consume a large amount of time. If, however, those four cases were performed in an ASC, turnover time was much shorter. It allowed me to place the patient safely in the recovery room, speak with her family, and dictate a procedure note before it was time to start the next case. This meant that those four cases could be accomplished by mid-morning and I could be off about other pursuits. Turnover time was reduced because the correct incentives were in place to make the facility run smoothly and safely.

The Need for Better Data on Physician Owners of ASCs

While I disagree with several of Gabel and colleagues' assertions, I do concur with their statements about the difficulty in interpretation of data because of the lack of public information about physician owners of ambulatory surgery centers. In fact, without this relevant data, any conclusion drawn becomes suspect – relying on broad generalities, or merely reinforcing preconceived notions. It is frequently hard to correct for observer bias. Additionally, the statements on the difference between Medicaid and Blue Cross Blue Shield – in other words, those ranging from the lowest to the highest payer – were somewhat confusing. As a clinician, why would I want to invest more of my most valuable commodity (time) to treat a patient for which my reimbursement is lowest? In the interest of precious time, it seems that the incentive for treating the Medicaid patient would be tilted toward the ASCs, so that it could be done more efficiently. Whenever I am confronted with a set of medical choices, my first default question is always, "Is it safe?" Secondly, I might consider, "What is the least complicated option for me and my patient?" And third, "What are the clinical as well as the business outcomes?" Thus, if I found myself recommending a procedure for a patient, and it could be safely performed in a surgery center, regardless of the amount of available compensation, the ease of scheduling and the rapidity of performance would tend to influence me toward the outpatient facility. There also might be a case to be made in terms of differentiation by specialties. Generalists such as gynecologists or general surgeons will typically have a broad mix of patients. Their diagnoses might reveal a different pattern than those among physicians who were more narrowly focused within a more well-defined specialty.

Differing Attitudes toward the Provision of Health Care

Finally, within the discussion section for this piece, perhaps the focus should not be on why the lowest reimbursement patients (Medicaid) were referred least often to an ASC. Instead, we should determine why Medicaid is the lowest payer. We should also explore what this says about those who want to expand the government's role in paying for health care. The paper talks about 11 a.m. on a Sunday morning. The statement is made that this might be the most segregated hour of the week. I am not certain about the source of that data, but I do wonder if there is a mindset of a segment of the population who believe that they should pay nothing for medical care versus those who search for an affordable option when hospital costs have increased to a level would preclude their use. The fact remains that both hospitals and ASCs are necessary for providing good, efficient, and cost-effective care in modern medicine. Physicians are more inherently aware of this fact than any other profession. Therefore, it is not surprising that they would want to provide these types of facilities or partner with their hospitals to provide these types of facilities, to provide the best possible care for their patients in an efficient and cost-effective manner. After all, it is patient care that really matters at the end of the day, and this begins and ends with doctors.

STATEMENT FOR THE RECORD: THE NATIONAL COMMUNITY PHARMACISTS ASSOCIATION (NCPA), UNITED STATES HOUSE OF REPRESENTATIVES ENERGY AND COMMERCE COMMITTEE SUBCOMMITTEE ON OVERSIGHT AND INVESTIGATIONS, HEARING: "EXAMINING THE IMPACT OF HEALTH CARE CONSOLIDATION" FEBRUARY 14, 2018

Chairman Harper, Ranking Member DeGette, and Members of the Subcommittee:

Thank you for conducting this hearing to explore consolidation in the health care industry and more important its effects on patients and consumers. In this statement, NCPA would like to present our thoughts on how the increased consolidation in the Pharmacy Benefit Manager (PBM) marketplace is contributing to higher consumer costs and impacting consumer choice when it comes to their pharmacy provider. PBMs are "middlemen" in the supply chain that determine formulary composition, pharmacy networks, and ultimately costs for consumers and plan sponsors, among other roles.

NCPA represents America's community pharmacists, including the owners of more than 22,000 independent community pharmacies. Together they represent an $80 billion health care marketplace and employ more than 250,000 individuals on a full or part-time basis. Independent community pharmacies are also typically located in traditionally underserved rural and urban communities, providing critical access to residents of these communities.

Concentrated PBM Marketplace

Due to mergers over the past several years, just three large companies now dominate the PBM market, and these three companies collect more than $200 billion a year to manage prescription services for insurance carriers covering 180 million Americans and government programs servicing about 110 million more.[111] In addition, the largest PBM has increased its profit per-adjusted prescription 500 percent since 2003.[112]

In fact, a 2017 report by the American Consumer Institute noted "because of recent mergers, the PBM market has increased in concentration, and that provides negotiating leverage which enables them to extract additional revenues and earnings."[113] The report further highlighted the market distortion between PBMs and pharmacies which has been exacerbated by consolidation, "[i]ncreased market concentration has allowed PBMs to become price-makers, and pharmacies as price-takers."[114]

Moreover, a 2015 hearing by the House Judiciary Committee Subcommittee on Regulatory Reform, Commercial and Antitrust Law raised additional concerns over consolidation in the PBM marketplace. Thomas Greaney, a Professor of Law at St. Louis University School of Law, testified at the hearing and suggested that it may be time for the FTC to review the PBM market and the effects of consolidation considering its previous decision to allow the merger of two of the largest PBMs, Express Scripts and Medco. At the same hearing, now FDA Commissioner, Scott

---

[111] *How 'price cutting' middlemen are making crucial drugs vastly more expensive, available at* http://www.latimes.com/business/hilzik/la-fi-hiltzik-pbm-drugs-20170611-story.html.
[112] Investor's Business Daily, Nov. 21, 2016, *available at* http://www.investors.com/politics/commentary/a-sick-calculation-about-prescription-drugs/.
[113] Pociask, Steve, *Pharmacy Benefit Managers: Market Power and Lack of Transparency*, p. 5, March 7, 2017, *available at* http://www.theamericanconsumer.org/2017/03/10882/.
[114] *Id.*

Gottlieb, voiced concerns over PBMs using their increased market power to capture revenue from other market participants. He noted this would be less concerning if it were easier for new PBMS to start up or smaller PBMs to grow, but he concluded, "[q]uite frankly I think the health plan consolidation will make it harder for smaller PBMs to continue to grow and will potentially give more market share to some of the existing large PBMs."[115]

Effects of PBM Consolidation on Consumers and Payers

A recent report from the White House Council of Economic Advisers noted the effects that PBM consolidation is playing in the marketplace stating that the three large PBMs account for 85 percent of the market, "which allows them to exercise undue market power against manufacturers and against the health plans and beneficiaries they are supposed to be representing, thus generating outsized profits for themselves."[116]

For large programs, including government-funded programs like Medicare Part D and the Federal Employee Health Benefits Program (FEHB), as well as large private employer-sponsored plans, there are few alternatives to these three PBMs that are large enough to manage such programs. Thus plan sponsors for these programs have limited choices. And while these three large PBMs may claim their size enables them to achieve market efficiencies, there is no requirement that these savings be passed along to plan sponsors and consumers. As the American Consumer Institute noted, "there is no market pressure for the PBMs to flow these savings through to sponsors or to consumers."[117] With patient out of pocket

---

[115] *The State of Competition in the Health Care Marketplace: The Patient Protection and Affordable Care Act's Impact on Competition: Hearing before the House Judiciary Subcommittee on Regulatory Reform, Commercial and Antitrust Law*, p. 120, Sept. 10, 2015, available at https://judiciary.house.gov/wp-content/uploads/2016/02/114-46_96053.pdf.

[116] The Council of Economic Advisors, *Reforming Biopharmaceutical Pricing at Home and Abroad*, p. 11, Feb. 2018, available at https://www.whitehouse.gov/wp-content/uploads/2017/11/CEA-Rx-White-Paper-Final2.pdf.

[117] Pociask, p.6.

costs and premiums continuing to rise, there is evidence to suggest that these savings are not, in fact, being passed on.

The market power PBMs exert also allows them to dictate contract terms to pharmacies, and in some cases exclude certain pharmacies from their networks altogether, limiting consumer choice. Community pharmacies routinely must agree to take it or leave it contracts. Such contracts often include blind price terms and other provisions that disadvantage community pharmacies and their patients. The PBMs also push plan sponsors to adopt plan designs that favor usage of a retail, mail order, or specialty pharmacies in which the PBM has an ownership interest. Thus consumers may find it difficult to fill their medication at their pharmacy of choice.

When they can, their pharmacy may be filling the medication at a loss due to the PBM's reimbursement formula. This conflict of interest must be addressed.

PBM Industry Largely Unregulated

Given the immense market influence that PBMs exert, one would expect these entities to be subject to the same type of comprehensive regulation that is currently required of commercial health insurers. However, PBMs are not subject to industry-wide regulation similar to what is generally required of commercial health insurers.

There are no federal laws or regulations that are specific to the PBM industry. Instead, PBMs face a patchwork of regulations at the state level that are designed to curtail some of the more onerous PBM business practices such as abusive PBM audits of pharmacies and requirements that PBMs update their maximum allowable cost (MAC) lists in a timely fashion. These MAC lists are used to determine pharmacy reimbursements for many generic medications and need to be updated regularly to reflect current market conditions. The PBMs routinely argue that federal laws such as ERISA preempt state initiatives to enforce regulations over them. At the same time, the PBMs aggressively assert that they are not subject to regulation under ERISA or other federal laws. As a result, the PBMs have capitalized on seemingly falling within a regulatory netherworld.

CVS Health -Aetna Inc. Merger and Its Potential Impact on Consumers

The pending merger between CVS Health and Aetna Inc. should be subject to strict scrutiny. While the merging parties claim they will create efficiencies in the marketplace, there are serious questions as to whether the purported savings with be passed on to plan sponsors and consumers. In addition, the merged entity with likely force or incentivize consumers to use providers associated with CVS Health and Aetna Inc. rather than the health providers of their own choosing, limiting consumer choice and potentially quality. Thus, a close examination of whether this acquisition will lead to higher drug prices and lower quality and fewer convenient pharmacy options for consumers is warranted.

Conclusion

The health care system continues to consolidate, especially when it comes to the PBM marketplace. More so, drug prices continue to increase, consumers are provided fewer choices where they can obtain their medications, payments to pharmacies are decreasing while costs to consumers are increasing and PBM profits continue to grow. Thus, any cost efficiencies obtained by the PBMs do not appear to be sufficiently trickling down to payers and consumers.

Members of this subcommittee should be concerned with this trend and how PBM actions are affecting taxpayer-funded programs given the fact that the federal government is the largest single payer of health care in the United States.[118] It is incumbent upon Congress to demand accountability to ensure a competitive marketplace that enables consumer choice by supporting common-sense legislative solutions.

GREG WALDEN, OREGON
CHAIRM AN

FRANK PALLONE, JR., NEW JERSEY
RANKING MEMBER

ONE HUNDRED FIFTEENTH CONGRESS, CONGRESS OF THE UNITED STATES, HOUSE OF REPRESENTATIVES, COMMITTEE ON ENERGY AND COMMERCE, MARCH 13, 2018

Dr. Martin S. Gaynor
E.J. Barone University Professor of Economics and Health Policy
Heinz College
Carnegie Mellon University
5000 Forbes Avenue
Pittsburgh, PA 15213

Dear Dr. Gaynor:

Thank you for appearing before the Subcommittee on Oversight and Investigations on February 14, 2018, to testify at the hearing entitled "Examining the Impact of Health Care Consolidation."

Pursuant to the Rules of the Committee on Energy and Commerce, the hearing record remains open for ten business days to permit Members to

---

[118] Troy, Tevi D., American Health Policy Institute, *How the Government As a Payer Shapes the Health Care Marketplace*, 2015.

submit additional questions for the record, which are attached. The format of your responses to these questions should be as follows: (1) the name of the Member whose question you are addressing, (2) the complete text of the question you are addressing in bold, and (3) your answer to that question in plain text.

To facilitate the printing of the hearing record, please respond to these questions with a transmittal letter by the close of business on Tuesday, March 27, 2018. Your responses should be mailed to Ali Fulling, Legislative Clerk, Committee on Energy and Commerce, 2125 Rayburn House Office Building, Washington, DC 20515 and e-mailed in Word format to Ali.Fulling@mail.house.gov.

Thank you again for your time and effort preparing and delivering testimony before the Subcommittee.

Sincerely,
Gregg Harper
Chairman
Subcommittee on Oversight and Investigations

cc: The Honorable Diana DeGette, Ranking Member, Subcommittee on Oversight and Investigations
Attachment

Additional Questions for the Record the Honorable Earl "Buddy" Carter

1. CMS data demonstrates a substantial migration of common procedures to higher-cost sites of service in hospital outpatient departments. For example, over the last several years (between 2010-2014), 6 percent of diagnostic colonoscopies have migrated into hospital outpatient departments that were previously performed in an ambulatory surgery center. (This costs both Medicare and its beneficiaries significantly more, as Medicare

spends $937 on diagnostic colonoscopies performed in hospital outpatient departments compared to $488 in ambulatory surgery centers. In addition, knee arthroscopy is down 16% in ASC and up 13% in HOPD.

This migration out of cheaper site-of-service is driven largely by hospital acquisition of physician practices, which in turn drives referrals. According to the Physician's Advocacy Institute, physician employment by hospitals grew by 49% between 2012 and 2015. What's more, for certain cardiology, orthopedic and gastroenterology services, hospital employment of physicians results in up to 27% higher costs for Medicare and 21% higher costs for patients.

a) Do you agree that the consolidation in healthcare, it's impact on physician referral practices and the migration of routine procedures to higher cost settings are related?
b) What can be done to ensure physicians offer Medicare beneficiaries and other patients access to the most efficient, high-quality and cost-effective care options?
c) Should ASC payment updates be tied to similar hospital outpatient facilities, so that independent physicians have a better chance to compete rather than becoming employed doctors?

Representative Yyvette Clarke

1. The current average price for a pair of eyeglasses is now around $400 per pair. Even as the price of eyeglasses is rising year-over-year, the eyewear industry is considering further consolidation. As it stands now, the market for eyeglass frames in the U.S. is largely dominated by one company, Luxottica, which owns and manufactures many of the top eyewear and sunglass brands. Notwithstanding its market dominance, Luxottica has proposed a merger with Essilor, a French company that controls around 70%

of the market share for lenses and the equipment to produce them. Together, a combined Luxottica-Essilor company would control and dominate the entire supply chain in the eyewear market.

a) How do you think this merger will impact the price of eyeglasses?
b) Do you think this merger will make it more difficult for smaller frame manufacturers, rival lens producers, and independent optometrists to compete and negotiate for market-based prices?

HEALTH CARE INDUSTRY CONSOLIDATION, RESPONSES TO QUESTIONS FROM THE COMMITTEE ON ENERGY AND COMMERCE OVERSIGHT AND INVESTIGATIONS SUBCOMMITTEE, U.S. HOUSE OF REPRESENTATIVES, BY MARTIN GAYNOR, E.J. BARONE UNIVERSITY PROFESSOR OF ECONOMICS AND HEALTH POLICY, HEINZ COLLEGE CARNEGIE MELLON UNIVERSITY, MARCH 23, 2018

1. Introduction

Below are my responses to questions from Members of the Committee on Energy and Commerce Oversight and Investigations Subcommittee, following the February 14, 2018 hearing "Examining the Impact of Health Care Consolidation."

2. Question from the Honorable Earl "Buddy" Carter

1. CMS data demonstrates a substantial migration of common procedures to higher-cost sites of service in hospital outpatient departments. For example, over the last several years (between 2010-2014), 6 percent of diagnostic colonoscopies have migrated

into hospital outpatient departments that were previously performed in an ambulatory surgery center. (This costs both Medicare and its beneficiaries significantly more, as Medicare spends $937 on diagnostic colonoscopies performed in hospital outpatient departments compared to $488 in ambulatory surgery centers. In addition, knee arthroscopy is down 16% in ASC and up 13% in HOPD.

This migration out of cheaper site-of-service is driven largely by hospital acquisition of physician practices, which in turn drives referrals. According to the Physicians Advocacy Institute, physician employment by hospitals grew by 49% between 2012 and 2015. Whats more, for certain cardiology, orthopedic and gastroenterology services, hospital employment of physicians results in up to 27% higher costs for Medicare and 21% higher costs for patients.

a) Do you agree that the consolidation in healthcare, its impact on physician referral practices and the migration of routine procedures to higher-cost settings are related?

The acquisition of physician practices by hospitals leads to more care being delivered in hospital settings (Capps et al., 2017; Koch et al., 2017; Dranove and Ody, 2016; Song et al., 2015) (although I am not aware of evidence specifically documenting a shift from ambulatory surgery centers to hospital outpatient departments as a result of such acquisitions).

There is direct evidence that hospital ownership of physician practices leads to more referrals to those (the owning) hospitals (Baker et al., 2016; Carlin et al., 2015), and that those hospitals are higher cost and lower quality (Baker et al., 2016). More generally, research has found that hospital ownership of physician practices is associated with higher spending and higher prices (Robinson and Miller, 2014; Baker et al., 2014; Neprash et al., 2015; Koch et al., 2017).

b) What can be done to ensure physicians offer Medicare beneficiaries and other patients access to the most efficient, high-quality and cost-effective care options?

Medicare should analyze how their payments are structured to see if the payments create unintended incentives that make treating patients in particular settings, locations, or facilities more financially rewarding than treating them in other settings, locations, or facilities. In particular, payments should be revised if necessary so that they do not favor any particular setting, facility, or location. Payments that reward more efficient, high quality, and cost effective care are desirable, but rewards should be based on the desired outcomes, as opposed to setting, facility, location, et'c.

c) Should ASC payment updates be tied to similar hospital outpatient facilities, so that independent physicians have a better chance to compete rather than becoming employed doctors?

It's desirable to have payments for providing the same service for patients of the same complexity and severity be equal, regardless of the setting. If patients can be provided with safe and high quality care in a lower cost setting then Medicare payments for all providers should be set at the level of the lower cost setting. For example, if patients can be provided with safe and high quality care in an ambulatory surgery center (ASC), and if the same treatment is cheaper in an ASC than in a hospital outpatient department, then Medicare payments should be set at the ASC level regardless of whether the treatment is provided in an ambulatory surgery center or a hospital outpatient department. The Medicare Payment Advisory Commission (Medpac) has outlined criteria under which hospital outpatient department payment rates could be aligned with ambulatory surgery center payment rates (Medicare Payment Advisory Commission, 2017).

3. Question from Representative Yvette Clarke

1. The current average price for a pair of eyeglasses is now around $400 per pair. Even as the price of eyeglasses is rising year-over-year, the eyewear industry is considering further consolidation. As it stands now, the market for eyeglass frames in the U.S. is largely dominated by one company, Lux-ottica, which owns and manufactures many of the top eyewear and sunglass brands. Notwithstanding its market dominance, Luxottica has proposed a merger with Essilor, a French company that controls around 70% of the market share for lenses and the equipment to produce them. Together, a combined Luxottica-Essilor company would control and dominate the entire supply chain in the eyewear market.

    a) How do you think this merger will impact the price of eyeglasses?

I do not have the information I would need to assess the likely impact of this merger. As a consequence, I do not have a personal opinion on the likely impact of the merger. However, the Federal Trade Commission (FTC) has reviewed the merger. The commissioners unanimously voted to close the investigation into the merger, because in their opinion the evidence did not indicate that the merger would substantially lessen competition (Federal Trade Commission, 2018). While I do not know all the particulars, I have a great deal of confidence in the FTC's ability to gather and analyze evidence and assess potential harms to competition.

    b) Do you think this merger will make it more difficult for smaller frame manufacturers, rival lens producers, and independent optometrists to compete and negotiate for market-based prices?

The FTC specifically addressed whether independent eye care professionals' ability to compete would be harmed by the merger. They concluded their ability to compete would not be harmed by the merger (Federal Trade Commission, 2018).

Bibliography

Baker, L., Bundorf, M., and Kessler, D. (2014). Vertical integration: Hospital ownership of physician practices is associated with higher prices and spending. *Health Affairs*, 33(5):756–763.

Baker, L. C., Bundorf, M. K., and Kessler, D. P. (2016). The effect of hospital/physician integration on hospital choice. *Journal of Health Economics*, 50:1–8.

Capps, C., Dranove, D., and Ody, C. (2017). The effect of hospital acquisitions of physician practices on prices and spending. unpublished manuscript, Northwestern University.

Carlin, C. S., Feldman, R., and Dowd, B. (2015). The impact of hospital acquisition of physician practices on referral patterns. *Health Economics*, 25(4):439–454.

Dranove, D. and Ody, C. (2016). Employed for higher pay? How Medicare facility fees affect hospital employment of physicians. unpublished manuscript, North-western University, https://faculty.kellogg.north western.edu/models/faculty/m_download_document.php?id=322.

Federal Trade Commission (2018). Statement of the Federal Trade Commission Concerning the Proposed Acquisition of Luxottica Group S.p.A. by Essilor International (Compagnie Generale d'Optique) S.A. FTC File No. 171-0060. https://www.ftc.gov/system/files/documents/closing_letters/nid/1710060commissionstatement.pdf.

Koch, T. G., Wendling, B. W., and Wilson, N. E. (2017). How vertical integration affects the quantity and cost of care for Medicare beneficiaries. *Journal of Health Economics*, 52:19 – 32.

Medicare Payment Advisory Commission (2017). Report to the Congress: Medicare payment policy. Technical report, Washington, D.C. Chapter 5, p. 142, http://www.medpac.gov/docs/default-source/reports/mar17_entirereport224610adfa9c665e80adff00009edf9c.pdf?sfvrsn=0.

Neprash, H., Chernew, M., Hicks, A., Gibson, T., and McWilliams, J. (2015). Association of financial integration between physicians and hospitals with commercial health care prices. *JAMA Internal Medicine*, 175(12):1932–1939.

Robinson, J. and Miller, K. (2014). Total expenditures per patient in hospital-owned and physician organizations in California. *JAMA*, 312(6):1663–1669.

Song, Z., Wallace, J., Neprash, H., McKellar, M., Chernew, M., and McWilliams, J. (2015). Medicare fee cuts and cardiologist-hospital integration. *JAMA Internal Medicine*, 175(7):1229–1231.

GREG WALDEN, OREGON
CHAIRMAN

FRANK PALLONE, JR., NEW JERSEY
RANKING MEMBER

ONE HUNDRED FIFTEENTH CONGRESS, CONGRESS OF THE UNITED STATES, HOUSE OF REPRESENTATIVES, COMMITTEE ON ENERGY AND COMMERCE, MARCH 13, 2018

Dr. Leemore S. Dafny
Bruce V. Rauner Professor of Business Administration
Harvard Business School
Morgan Hall 247
Soldiers Field Road
Boston, MA 02163

Dear Dr. Dafny:

Thank you for appearing before the Subcommittee on Oversight and Investigations on February 14, 2018, to testify at the hearing entitled "Examining the Impact of Health Care Consolidation."

Pursuant to the Rules of the Committee on Energy and Commerce, the hearing record remains open for ten business days to permit Members to submit additional questions for the record, which are attached. The format of your responses to these questions should be as follows: (1) the name of the Member whose question you are addressing, (2) the complete text of the question you are addressing in bold, and (3) your answer to that question in plain text.

To facilitate the printing of the hearing record, please respond to these questions with a transmittal letter by the close of business on Tuesday, March 27, 2018. Your responses should be mailed to Ali Fulling, Legislative Clerk, Committee on Energy and Commerce, 2125 Rayburn House Office Building, Washington, DC 20515 and e-mailed in Word format to Ali.Fulling@mail.house.gov.

Thank you again for your time and effort preparing and delivering testimony before the Subcommittee.

Gregg Harper Chairman
Subcommittee on Oversight and Investigations

cc: The Honorable Diana DeGette, Ranking Member, Subcommittee on Oversight and Investigations

ATTACHMENT-ADDITIONAL QUESTIONS FOR THE RECORD

The Honorable Michael C. Burgess

1. You write in your 2016 article entitled "Health Care Needs Real Competition" that continually improving electronic health record interoperability across delivery systems has major implications for competition. Can you explain the role that electronic health records and data could play in the competitiveness of the health care market?

The Honorable Yyvette Clarke

1. The current average price for a pair of eyeglasses is now around $400 per pair. Even as the price of eyeglasses is rising year-over-year, the eyewear industry is considering fm1her consolidation. As it stands now, the market for eyeglass frames in the U.S. is largely dominated by one company, Luxottica, which owns and manufactures many of the top eyewear and sunglass brands. Notwithstanding its market dominance, Luxottica has proposed a merger with Essilor, a French company that controls around 70% of the market share for lenses and the equipment to produce them. Together, a combined Luxottica-Essilor company would control and dominate the entire supply chain in the eyewear market.

    a) How do you think this merger will impact the price of eyeglasses?
    b) Do you think this merger will make it more difficult for smaller frame manufacturers, rival lens producers, and independent optometrists to compete and negotiate for market-based prices?

GREG WALDEN, OREGON, CHAIRMAN
FRANK PALLONE, JR., NEW JERSEY, RANKING MEMBER

ONE HUNDRED FIFTEENTH CONGRESS, CONGRESS OF THE UNITED STATES, HOUSE OF REPRESENTATIVES, COMMITTEE ON ENERGY AND COMMERCE, MARCH 13, 2018

Dr. Kevin A. Schulman, Professor of Medicine
Visiting Scholar, Harvard Business School
Duke University, P.O. Box 17969 Durham, NC 27715

Dear Dr. Schulman:

Thank you for appearing before the Subcommittee on Oversight and Investigations on February 14, 2018, to testify at the hearing entitled "Examining the Impact of Health Care Consolidation."

Pursuant to the Rules of the Committee on Energy and Commerce, the hearing record remains open for ten business days to permit Members to submit additional questions for the record, which are attached. The format of your responses to these questions should be as follows: (I) the name of the Member whose question you are addressing, (2) the complete text of the question you are addressing in bold, and (3) your answer to that question in plain text.

To facilitate the printing of the hearing record, please respond to these questions with a transmittal letter by the close of business on Tuesday, March 27, 2018. Your responses should be mailed to Ali Fulling, Legislative Clerk, Committee on Energy and Commerce, 2125 Rayburn House Office Building, Washington, DC 20515 and e-mailed in Word format to Ali.Fu lling@mail.house.gov.

Thank you again for your time and effort preparing and delive ring testimony before the Subcommittee.

Sincerely,
Gregg Harper
Chairman
Subcommittee on Oversight and Investigations
   cc: The Honorable Diana DeGette, Ranking Member, Subcommittee on Oversight and Investigations Attachment
Attachment

Additional Questions for the Record

The Honorable Yvvettc Clarke
1. The current average price for a pair of eyeglasses is now around $400 per pair. Even as the price of eyeglasses is rising year-over-

year, the eyewear industry is considering further consolidation. As it stands now, the market for eyeglass frames in the U.S. is largely dominated by one company, Luxottica, which owns and manufactures many of the top eyewear and sunglass brands. Notwithstanding its market dominance, Luxottica has proposed a merger with Essilor, a French company that controls around 70% of the market share for lenses and the equipment to produce them. Together, a combined Luxottica-Essilor company would control and dominate the entire supply chain in the eyewear market.

a) How do you think this merger will impact the price of eyeglasses?

b) Do you think this merger will make it more difficult for smaller frame manufacturers, rival lens producers, and independent optometrists to compete and negotiate for market-based prices?

ADDITIONAL QUESTION FOR THE RECORD, KEVIN A. SCHULMAN, MD, PROFESSOR OF MEDICINE DUKE UNIVERSITY DURHAM, NC, VISITING SCHOLAR HARVARD BUSINESS SCHOOL, BOSTON, MA, COMMITTEE ON ENERGY AND COMMERCE SUBCOMMITTEE ON OVERSIGHT AND INVESTIGATIONS, MARCH 21, 2018

Questions from the Honorable Yvette Clarke

1. The current average price for a pair of eyeglasses is now around $400 per pair. Even as the price of eyeglasses is rising, the eyewear industry is considering further consolidation. As it stands now, the market for eyeglass frames in the US is largely dominated by one company, Luxottica, which owns and manufactures many of the top eyewear and sunglass brands. Notwithstanding it's

market dominance, Luxottica has proposed a merger with Essilor, a French company that controls around 70% of the market share for lenses and the equipment to produce them. Together, a combined Luxottica-Essilor company would control and dominate the entire supply chain in the eyewear market.

Response:

Our panel did not address consolidation in the eyewear marketplace, and there is little medical literature addressing this market.

In the business literature, reports suggest that Luxottica holds an estimated 60-80% market share of the retail eyewear market.[119] As you suggest, this market position includes control over retail outlets (including Lenscrafters, Pearle Vision Center, and Sunglass Hut, and Sears Optical[120]), and eyewear brands (28 including Ray Ban and Oakley[121]). Essilor controls 13 brands of eyeglass lenses and eyewear products.[122]

However, there are reasons to believe that the retail market may not be as concentrated as these data suggest. One analysis reports a 2016 market share of eyewear sales of 45.8% for independent outlets, 26.6% for chains, 16.3% for mass merchandisers, 4.5% for department stores, 4.2% for internet sales, and 6.8% other retailers, with modest increasing share since 2013 for independent outlets and internet sales, and modest decreasing share for chains, mass merchandisers, and department stores since 2013.[123]

The proposed merger of Luxottica-Essilor was cleared by the US Federal Trade Commission on March 1, 2018.[124]

a. How do you think this merger will impact the price of eyeglasses?

---

[119] https://www.gurufocus.com/news/318329/is-competition-in-the-eyewear-segment-preying-over-luxotticas-bottom-line.
[120] http://www.luxottica.com/en/retail-brands.
[121] http://www.luxottica.com/en/eyewear-brands.
[122] https://www.essilor.com/en/brands-and-solutions/our-brands/.
[123] https://www.statista.com/statistics/256255/sales-share-of-the-frame-market-for-eyewear-in-the-us-by-retail-chain/.
[124] https://www.essilor.com/en/medias/press-releases/proposed-combination-essilor-luxottica-receives-clearance-us-federal-trade-commission-without-conditions/.

Response:
The economics literature provides a sophisticated assessment of the potential implications of such a merger. Consumers may benefit depending on the pricing decisions of the integrated firm (highlighted below), but as with any economics model there are significant caveats to this result.

"Vertical externalities: A classical explanation for vertical integration is as a response to inefficiencies that arise when there is market power in both the upstream and downstream markets.[125] This in turn implies that market prices will be greater than the marginal cost of production in both upstream and downstream markets as firms exercise market power. The polar case is one where there is a pure monopoly upstream ("manufacturing") and another pure monopoly downstream ("retailing") and where the upstream monopoly has all of the bargaining power over the price that will be charged for goods or services sold by the upstream firm to the downstream firm. The monopoly at the upstream "manufacturing" level has a marginal production cost c and seeks to charge a monopoly input price PM > c to the downstream firm. The downstream "retail" monopoly takes the price PM as its input cost and exercises its monopoly power by charging a retail price PRM > PM. The upstream monopoly has added a monopoly markup to its production costs and then the downstream monopoly has added another markup to the price it pays to the upstream firm for its inputs. This phenomenon is known as double-marginalization. When making its pricing decisions, the downstream monopoly ignores (because it does not see) the actual costs of production incurred by the upstream firm. This behavior of the independent monopolies results in aggregate profits that are smaller than they would be in the firms set prices so as to maximize their joint profits. It also leads to higher prices downstream than would maximize the joint profits if the upstream and downstream firms. Tirole refers to the failure of the downstream firm to take upstream production costs into account as a vertical externality (Tirole, 1988, Chapter 4).

If we assume that vertical integration is costless, the aggregate profits of the two monopolies will increase if they merge since the distortion

---

[125] Market power as that term is used in economic theory. Firms face downward sloping demand curves and are not pure price takers. There need not be supra-normal profits in equilibrium, however."

from double marginalization will disappear. The integrated firm will set the profit maximizing downstream monopoly price properly taking into account the actual costs of production at the upstream level. Moreover, prices charged to consumers will fall and, as a result, consumers are made better off by vertical integration. This is the classic example of the maxim that a single monopoly is better than a chain of monopolies.

c) Do you think this merger will make it more difficult for smaller frame manufacturers, rival lens producers, and independent optometrists to compete and negotiate for market-based prices?

Response:

As an independent firm, Essilor, the lens manufacturer, would want to maintain a competitive retail market for it's products to ensure that it had negotiating leverage and marketing options if retailer Luxottica tried to exert pricing pressure on Essilor, although as the literature suggests Essilor could still exert it's market power in setting the price for their products.

As an integrated firm, there may be significant pricing advantages offered to their internal retail customers compared with smaller volume external retailers. This could serve as a barrier to entry to the retail market and could result in increased prices for consumers. Further efforts by the merged firm to continue the horizontal integration of the retail or lens market should carefully consider the market power and marketing and pricing activities of the merged firm.

The one caveat to this concern is the emergence of a novel, vertically-integrated rival, Warby Parker.[126] This start-up has spawned a more competitive market for eyewear using an internet-based retailing model (now supplemented by retail stores), and suggests that barriers to entry into the eyewear space are not insurmountable for novel entrants. Their success should impose significant price pressure on existing retailers in the market,

---

[126] https://www.forbes.com/sites/stevedenning/2016/03/23/whats-behind-warby-parkers-success/#2deb3ced411a.

and on the merged Luxottica-Essilor entity. However, this price pressure will only exist if consumers learn to shop for eyewear products across brands and retail outlets. It also requires consumers to have access to their lens prescriptions so that they can shop for the best prices on their eyewear products.

Many of the existing independent retailers in this market may feel increasing pressure on their margins from the expanded market power of existing retail chains as a result of the Luxottica-Essilor merger and from the emergence of a new, internet-based eyewear retail channel.

In: Health Care Consolidation ...
Editor: Dominik Vogel

ISBN: 978-1-53616-870-9
© 2019 Nova Science Publishers, Inc.

Chapter 2

EXAMINING THE EFFECTIVENESS OF THE INDIVIDUAL MANDATE UNDER THE AFFORDABLE CARE ACT

TUESDAY, JANUARY 24, 2017

U.S. HOUSE OF REPRESENTATIVES, COMMITTEE ON WAYS AND MEANS, SUBCOMMITTEE ON OVERSIGHT,
Washington, DC.

The Subcommittee met, pursuant to call, at 2:26 p.m., in Room 1100, Longworth House Office Building, Hon. Vern Buchanan [Chairman of the Subcommittee] presiding.

[The advisory announcing the hearing follows:]

CHAIRMAN BUCHANAN ANNOUNCES HEARING ON EXAMINING THE EFFECTIVENESSOF THE INDIVIDUAL MANDATE

Under the Affordable Care Act

House Committee on Ways and Means Subcommittee on Oversight Chairman Vern Buchanan (R-FL) today announced that the Subcommittee will hold a hearing on Examining the Effectiveness of the Individual Mandate under the Affordable Care Act. The hearing will take place immediately following a brief Subcommittee Organizational Meeting on Tuesday, January 24, 2017 at 2:00 PM in Room 1100 of the Longworth House Office Building.

In view of the limited time to hear witnesses, oral testimony at this hearing will be from invited witnesses only. However, any individual or organization may submit a written statement for consideration by the Committee and for inclusion in the printed record of the hearing.

Details for Submission of Written Comments

Please Note: Any person(s) and/or organization(s) wishing to submit written comments for the hearing record must follow the appropriate link on the hearing page of the Committee website and complete the informational forms. From the Committee homepage, http://waysandmeans.house.gov, select "Hearings." Select the hearing for which you would like to make a submission, and click on the link entitled, "Click here to provide a submission for the record. Once you have followed the online instructions, submit all requested information. ATTACH your submission as a Word document, in compliance with the formatting requirements listed below, by the close of business on Tuesday, February 7, 2017. For questions, or if you encounter technical problems, please call (202) 225-3625.

Formatting Requirements

The Committee relies on electronic submissions for printing the official hearing record. As always, submissions will be included in the record according to the discretion of the Committee. The Committee will not alter the content of your submission, but we reserve the right to format it according to our guidelines. Any submission provided to the Committee by a witness, any materials submitted for the printed record, and any written comments in response to a request for written comments must conform to the guidelines listed below. Any submission not in compliance with these guidelines will not be printed, but will be maintained in the Committee files for review and use by the Committee.

All submissions and supplementary materials must be submitted in a single document via email, provided in Word format and must not exceed a total of 10 pages. Witnesses and submitters are advised that the Committee relies on electronic submissions for printing the official hearing record.

All submissions must include a list of all clients, persons and/or organizations on whose behalf the witness appears. The name, company, address, telephone, and fax numbers of each witness must be included in the body of the email. Please exclude any personal identifiable information in the attached submission.

Failure to follow the formatting requirements may result in the exclusion of a submission All submissions for the record are final.

The Committee seeks to make its facilities accessible to persons with disabilities. If you are in need of special accommodations, please call 202-225-1721 or 202-226-3411 TTD/TTY in advance of the event (four business days notice is requested). Questions with regard to special accommodation needs in general (including availability of Committee materials in alternative formats) may be directed to the Committee as noted above.

Note: All Committee advisories and news releases are available at http://www.waysandmeans, house.gov/.

Chairman BUCHANAN. The Subcommittee will come to order.

Welcome to the Ways and Means Subcommittee Oversight hearing on Examining the Effectiveness of the Individual Mandate Under the Affordable Care Act. My focus today is on affordability.

In Florida, 65 percent of our counties only have one carrier offering insurance to individuals in 2017. The State went from eight carriers in 2014. Today, we have five carriers, almost half, in 2017. In Manatee and Sarasota Counties, two counties I represent in my district, individuals went from being able to choose from among three different providers down to two. This happened in just a single year. In addition to less options to choose from, the average monthly premium Floridians enjoyed under the ACA increased by 19 percent this past year, according to the Florida Office of Insurance Regulation.

Let me pause and look back 4 years ago when the Affordable Care Act was just beginning to be implemented in 2013. Then, the HHS secretary released a report stating the goal of Affordable Healthcare Act is to increase competition and transparency in the markets for individuals and small group insurance leading to higher quality, more affordable products. Fast forward 4 years later, 2017, what we are seeing not only in Florida but across the country is a decrease in competition, an increase in premium costs. This increase cannot continue. It is not sustainable.

We are here today to understand why the individual mandate, which today I think those fees that we are paying in over $3 billion was a key component. The ACA is failing to stabilize the health insurance marketplace. This discussion is important not so that members on our side of the aisle or the other side of the aisle can score political points, but that, so we can focus on the facts. We need facts because there are real people's lives that are being impacted.

When I talk to people in my district, it is clear to me that they are struggling. Although I mentioned some statewide and county- level statistics, those numbers touch the lives of real people in Florida in terms of Florida families. We cannot stand idly by as health insurance under the Affordable Care Act becomes less and less affordable for our constituents. I hope this hearing serves as the first step to fixing what is broken. I look forward to listening to our witnesses and learning from the past so that we can develop better solutions for the future.

I now yield to the distinguished Ranking Member Mr. Lewis for the purpose of an opening statement.

Mr. LEWIS. Again, Mr. Chairman, thank you. I want to thank you again and congratulate you on your new role as chairman of the Oversight Subcommittee.

The two Democratic Members of the Subcommittee have now arrived. They didn't get lost in the tunnel. So they are here. Joe Crowley of New York and Danny Davis of Illinois.

Mr. Chairman, I hope we can continue our tradition of strong oversight of the Administration as we have in past Congresses. I would also like to thank each witness for being here this afternoon.

Let me begin by saying what I have said at countless other hearings. The Affordable Care Act works. It works. Now, I want to be crystal clear for the record. The topic of today's hearing is a Republican idea. In fact, Governor Romney called it the ultimate conservative idea because it was based in personal responsibility. The individual mandate became a core part of the health care law. There is not a family in this country that has not been touched by sickness or injury. By sickness or injury.

I have said it before and I will say it again. I believe in my heart of hearts that health care is a basic human right. It is not a privilege for the wealthy. It should not be reserved for the people that insurance companies have decided worthy of the risk.

This Committee has a mission, an obligation, and a mandate to think of those that have been left out and left behind. We cannot forget the 100 million Americans with preexisting conditions. We cannot forget the struggle of those people whose care costs more than the insurance limit. We cannot forget the seniors in the doughnut hole who were unable to afford their medicine.

I know that we can come together to make health care more affordable, more accessible for every person in our great country. I speak for the members on this side of the aisle who are ready to do the good work, the people's work.

We must be mindful not to harm the marketplaces where Americans buy insurance. We must protect children from being kicked off of their parents' plan. We must ensure that a woman is not charged more simply because she is a woman.

Mr. Chairman, today we face a moral issue. In the coming weeks and months, we should come together to improve the law and not destroy it. At stake are not just the detail of policy but the fundamental principles of justice and the very character like our great Nation.

Thank you, Mr. Chairman. And I yield back.

Chairman BUCHANAN. Thank you, Mr. Lewis.

Without objection, other Members' opening statements will be made part of the record.

Today's witness panel includes three experts. First, John Graham is a senior fellow at the National Center for Policy Analysis. Tom Miller is a resident fellow at the American Enterprise Institute. And finally, Dr. John E. McDonough is a professor of practice at the Department of Health Policy and Management at Harvard TH Chan School of Public Health.

The Subcommittee has received your written statements and they will be all made part of the formal hearing record. You will each have 5 minutes to deliver your oral remarks. We will begin with Mr. Graham. You may begin when you are ready.

STATEMENT OF JOHN R. GRAHAM, SENIOR FELLOW AT THE NATIONAL CENTER FOR POLICY ANALYSIS

Mr. GRAHAM. Thank you, sir.

Chairman Buchanan, Ranking Member Lewis, my name is John R. Graham of the National Center for Policy Analysis. I will take my short time today to emphasize some of the commentary I brought up in my written comments, which I have already submitted to you and which I drafted before President Trump issued his executive order, which I think makes the individual mandate of even more pressing concern.

Will it be enforced by the next HHS secretary? If it is not enforced, will it cause ObamaCare to collapse? Or perhaps some of us might say collapse more or faster than we have seen it collapsing already.

Politically, it is very easy to go after the individual mandate. It is the least popular part of ObamaCare. However, it counterbalances the most popular part of ObamaCare, the protection against being underwritten for preexisting conditions.

I think my message today could be worry not. Although the individual mandate is also—is bad politics, I would also assert it is bad economics or at least weak economics. Now, this is a very different message than we have heard for many, many years. It is true that it can properly be characterized as a conservative idea. And the high water mark of that was what we call RomneyCare in the Massachusetts health reform. The idea which is meant to appeal to conservatives is that this is—demonstrates individual responsibility. We have a problem that hospitals' emergency rooms are jammed with patients who are not paying their bills, and so we have an uncompensated care crisis. Fair enough.

Further, if people are encouraged to buy more insurance, they are more likely to get preventative and timely care and not have to go to the emergency room in the first place. Well, that would be fine. But the reality on the ground is it would only work if the mandate or the uninsured crisis was concentrated among high-income households. If it was folks like Bill Gates or Warren Buffett who were crowding the emergency rooms. I am sorry. I should update that given the current Administration. Peter Thiel or Sheldon Adelson were crowding the emergency rooms. But they are not. It is low-income people who are largely uninsured. They cannot bear to pay the fee or tax or penalty or whatever we want to call it for violating the mandate.

So although it is appealing to conservatives to think that this imposes individual responsibility, in fact what its real effect is to give cover to significant growth in government spending and government programs, which is fine in some people's minds but not for conservative minds, I would suggest.

Now, whatever we want to call it—the law, as you know, calls it a penalty. CMS healthcare.gov now calls it a fee. But whatever we want to call it, it is inefficient in a very mechanical sense. A recent memo from the Internal Revenue Service points out that 6- 1/2 million people paid the fine in 2015, but 12.7 million were exempted for various reasons. Again, emphasizing the point that most people whom you think you are affecting with a mandate cannot afford to pay it.

How much was raised from the mandate? $3 billion. Now, to me that sounds like a lot of money. But as you know, in the health care system that is nothing. We spent $3.2 trillion on health care in this country in 2015. If we compare the Congressional Budget Office score to—about ObamaCare, the Affordable Care Act in 2010 versus the update in March 2016, it shows there is a slight reduction in anticipated revenue from the tax or penalty from the people who do not obey the mandate. But this is not because more people are getting private coverage and exercising their responsibility.

In the original CBO score, the CBO estimated, this is back in 2010, that the Affordable Care Act would leave 22 million uninsured in 2016 through 2019. Recently, that has been upped to 27 million. Those with employer-based coverage, according to the original estimate, was 163 million. In the new estimate, it is down to 159 million. Sorry. Down to 152 million.

In 2010, the Congressional Budget Office estimated ObamaCare exchanges would enroll 21 million people in 2016, and we know where that has gone, increasing to 24 million in 2019. It is down to an estimate of 20 million people in 2019 under the current law, according to the latest CBO estimate.

Who is getting insured? It is Medicaid. And the Medicaid dependency, the estimates according to the CBO, have gone up by about one-third. So the coverage through ObamaCare is not through enforcing any kind of individual mandate. It is through more government dependency on Medicaid, which is costing us far more than we are getting from an individual mandate.

Chairman BUCHANAN. Thank you.
[The prepared statement of Mr. Graham follows:]
"Obamacare's Individual Mandate is Economically inefficient and Does Not Improve Access to Health Care"
Statement of John R. Graham
Senior Fellow National Center for Policy Analysis
Committee on Ways and Means
Subcommittee on Oversight "Examining the Effectiveness of the Individual Mandate under the ACA"

Chairman Buchanan, Ranking Member Lewis, and Members of the Committee, I am John R. Graham, Senior Fellow at the National Center for Policy Analysis, a nonprofit, nonpartisan public policy research organization dedicated to developing and promoting private alternatives to government regulation and control, solving problems by relying on the strength of the competitive, entrepreneurial private sector. I welcome the opportunity to share my views and look forward to your questions.

The individual mandate is Obamacare's least popular feature. It was the subject of the 2012 lawsuit asserting Obamacare was unconstitutional: Never before had the federal government forced any resident to buy a good or service from a private business. The people lost that argument. Nevertheless, Republicans have pledged to eliminate the individual mandate. This commitment remains good politics. Perhaps counterintuitively, it is also good economics.

According to last November's Kaiser Family Foundation Tracking Poll, only 35 percent of respondents have a favorable view of the individual mandate. The proportion drops to just 21 percent among Republicans, and just 16 percent among Trump supporters[1].

However, getting rid of the individual mandate also poses a political dilemma: It balances a very popular provision of Obamacare. Recall the theory of the individual mandate is to prevent freeriding: Americans should

---

[1] Kaiser Health Tracking Poll: November 2016," The Henry H. Kaiser Family Foundation, December 1, 2016. Available at http://kff.org/health-costs/poll-finding/kaiser-health-tracking-poll-november-2016/.

be responsible for maintaining continuous health coverage so they do not become a burden on taxpayers when they become sick.

If you bought a house and did not invest in homeowner's insurance, few citizens would urge the government to require insurers to issue you a policy after your house was destroyed by fire. We all understand the market for homeowner's insurance could not function under such a law.

However, we seem to have a blind spot with respect to this problem when it comes to health insurance. In the same poll, 69 percent of respondents support prohibiting insurers from denying coverage because of a person's medical history. The proportion is 63 percent among Republicans, and 60 percent among Trump supporters.

This appears to support the academic economic argument for the individual mandate alongside a means-tested tax credit for buying health insurance: Without them, people will wait until they become sick to buy health insurance. President Obama and his allies came to accept the academic argument without recognizing its political costs. Further, as was discussed back in 2009 and 2010, the individual mandate has been described as a "conservative" or even "Republican" idea. Championed by an influential conservative think tank, it was integral to Governor Mitt Romney's 2006 health reform in Massachusetts. Characterized as a feature of individual responsibility, the individual mandate would give bipartisan political cover to a significant growth of government spending and control over health insurance.

Of course, history shows it did not achieve that cover. Fortunately, evidence show the individual mandate is also bad economics, despite academic claims. Whatever we label the punishment for disobeying the mandate - a "fine" or a "tax" - it is a very, very inefficient way to finance health care. Although the Centers for Medicare & Medicaid Services refers to a "fee," the Affordable Care Act names it a "penalty," which is the word used in this testimony).

In many other insurance markets, politicians do not become overly concerned with the risk of free-riders. If a person does not buy homeowner's insurance, and his house burns down, most would agree he was irresponsible. However, no politician would commit taxpayers to rebuild and refurnish his house. Health care is different. Americans receive treatment, especially at hospitals, whether we can pay or not. The argument from individual responsibility claims some people do not buy health insurance voluntarily, then get rushed to hospitals' emergency rooms. The hospitals suffer a burden of so-called uncompensated care, which the text of the Affordable Care Act asserted added one thousand dollars to the average premium of insured people (because hospitals raise charges to cover uncompensated care).

If the government imposes an individual mandate to maintain health insurance or pay a penalty, there will be a significant reduction in uncompensated care, and this hidden tax should come off our premiums. Also, being insured should increase the likelihood of being treated by a doctor early in the development of a problem, and avoiding the emergency department altogether.

Unfortunately, the consequences of the individual mandate are quite different in the real world. The only way the individual mandate would solve the problem of uncompensated care is if high-income people were the ones receiving uncompensated care. They are not. It is lowincome people who dominate the uninsured. So, increasing the number of people with health insurance requires far more tax credits flowing out to subsidize their coverage than revenues from penalties. This drives health costs up.

The net cash flows are complicated because neither health insurers nor hospitals and other providers would tolerate tax credits being paid to individuals directly. This would impose significant credit risk throughout the health system. As a result, the Affordable Care Act pays tax credits to insurers, which reduces net premiums due from beneficiaries.

Nevertheless, a recent report from the IRS demonstrates the confusion[2]. For 2015:

---

[2] John A. Koskinen, letter to Congress regarding 2016 tax filings related to Affordable Care Act provisions, Internati Revenue Service, January 9, 2017. Available at https://www.irs.gov/pub/newsroom/commissionerletteracafilingseason.pdf.

- According to forms submitted with individuals' tax returns, about 5.8 million taxpayers received advance payments of premium tax credits.
- However, according to forms submitted to the IRS by Obamacare's exchanges, 7.3 million taxpayers received advances.
- The IRS figures the difference (about 1.5 million people) comprises taxpayers who have not filed the appropriate form with their tax returns.
- About 2.4 million taxpayers claimed more tax credit in their tax return than they had received in advance.
- About 3.3 million taxpayers reported they had received too much in advance and had to refund some. The total was $2.9 billion.

As for the individual mandate:

- About 12.7 million taxpayers filed for an exemption from the mandate. (There are a number of grounds for exemption, including self-declared "hardship").
- About 6.5 million taxpayers reported a total of $3.0 billion in penalties due for not maintaining coverage.

Recall U.S. health spending in 2015 was $3.2 trillion, so the penalties comprise an utterly trivial share of health care financing[3]. Even within Obamacare, revenue from penalties were never very significant. According to the Congressional Budget Office's original score of the Affordable Care Act, the individual mandate was estimated to raise $17 billion over ten years (2010 through 2019), only 2 percent of Obamacare's $1 trillion dollar source of funds[4]. In the March 2016 baseline, the CBO updated its

---

[3] National Health Expenditures 2015 Highlights, Centers for Medicare & Medicaid Services, December 6, 2016. Available at https://www.cms.gov/Research-Statistics-Data-and-Systems/Statistics-Trends-andReports/NationalHealthExpendData/downloads/highlights.pdf.

[4] "Cost estimate for the amendment in the nature of a substitute for H.R. 4872, incorporating a proposed manager's amendment," Congressional Budget Office, March 20, 2010. Available at https://www.cbo.gov/publication/21351.

Examining the Effectiveness of the Individual Mandate ... 193

estimate of revenue from penalties.[5] For the four years included in both the 2010 and 2016 estimates (2016 through 2019), the estimate dropped one fifth from $15 billion to $12 billion.

However, this is not because more people are expected to pay for their own insurance. On the contrary, more are expected to be uninsured or fall into Medicaid, a welfare program fully funded by taxpayers. The changes are significant:

- In 2010, CBO estimated Obamacare would leave 22 million uninsured in 2016 through 2019. In 2016, CBO estimated Obamacare will leave 27 million uninsured through 2019 - an increase of almost one quarter.
- In 2010, CBO estimated Obamacare would leave 163 million with employer-based health benefits in 2016 and 159 million in 2019. In 2016, CBO estimated Obamacare will leave only 155 million with employer-based plans. The number will decrease to 152 million in 2019.
- In 2010, CBO estimated Obamacare exchanges would enroll 21 million people in 2016, increasing to 24 million in 2019. In 2016, CBO estimated Obamacare's exchanges will enroll only 13 million people this year, and 20 million in 2019.
- In 2010, CBO estimated Obamacare would result in 52 million Americans remaining or falling into dependency on Medicaid or the Children's Health Insurance Program, the welfare programs jointly funded by state and federal governments that subsidizes lowincome households' health care, in 2016. CBO estimated that figure would drop slightly to 51 million in 2019. In 2016, CBO estimated 68 million will be dependent on the program this year through 2019 - an increase of almost one third in the welfare caseload.

---

[5] "Federal Subsidies for Health Insurance Coverage for People under Age 65: Tables from CBO's March 2016 Baseline," Congressional Budget Office, March 2016. Available at https://www.cbo.gov/sites/default/files/recurringdata/51298-2016-03-healthinsurance.pdf.

If there is any positive to this news, it is that Obamacare's exchange spending will be less than initially estimated. Because the estimated number of people enrolling in Obamacare's exchanges has been cut almost in half, the estimate of taxpayer dollars handed out to insurers in the exchanges has also been reduced. The initial estimate for the 2016-2019 period was $394 billion, which has been dialed back to $243 billion in the March 2016 update.

Of course, those 16 million more welfare dependents will be a burden on taxpayers. Because of differences in the way CBO reports Obamacare's effect on Medicaid and the CHIP in its 2010 and March 2016 estimates, it is not easy to calculate the change in Medicaid and CHIP spending due to Obamacare.

Nevertheless, this month's CBO estimate alone indicates $64 billion, almost one quarter of the $279 billion the federal government will spend on Medicaid and SCHIP this year, is due to Obamacare's Medicaid expansion.[6]

This is broadly reminiscent of the experience of Massachusetts' 2006 reform. In its 2007-2008 Progress Report, the state noted 97,000 uninsured residents (58 percent of the uninsured) were assessed a (very small) penalty in 2007.[7] However, of the 434,000 who became newly insured through March 2008, 72,000 were enrolled in the fully subsidized MassHealth program and 176,000 in the partially subsidized Commonwealth Care. Although, a majority of enrollees in Commonwealth Care did not actually pay any premium. The proportion paying premium increased from 20 percent in August 2007 to 42 percent in 2013 the last year before Obamacare.[8] For most beneficiaries, Commonwealth Care was wholly welfare.

---

[6] In 2010, CBO's total estimate of 52 million dependents in 2016 comprised a baseline of 35 million plus 17 million more due to Obamacare's expansion. This month, CBO's estimate of 68 million comprised a baseline of 57 million dependents if Obamacare had not passed, plus 11 million due to Obamacare's expansion.

[7] "Massachusetts Health Care Reform: 2007/2008 Progress Report," Commonwealth Connector, 2008, page 8. Available at https://www.mahealthconnector.org/wp-content/uploads/progressreports/2007_2008ProgressReport.pdf.

[8] "Report to the Massachusetts Legislature, Implementation of the Health Care Reform Law, Chapter 58, 20062008," The Massachusetts Health Care Connector Authority, October 2,

State and federal spending attributable to Massachusetts health reform almost doubled from $1.0 billion in 2006 to $1.9 billion in 2011. The reform drove up health spending. Hospitals' emergency department use increased by 17 percent in the two years after the reform was implemented.[9]

The reform also gave the insurance commissioner political power to dictate insurance premiums. The commissioner refused 235 of 276 rate hikes for April 2010 and demanded that plans rebate premiums that had already been paid.[10] The result is that Massachusetts' health plans hemorrhaged cash, and a senior regulator described the situation as a "train wreck."[11]

Similarly, the average Obamacare premium hike for 2017 was 25 percent, demonstrating an individual mandate does not reduce premium growth by making everyone pay their fair share.[12] A friendly 2014 analysis published by the U.S. Department of Health & Human Services estimated Obamacare would reduce uncompensated care costs by $5.7 billion that year.[13] However, Medicaid and Obamacare tax credits cost the federal government alone $38 billion in 2014. It makes no sense to spend $38 billion to save $5.7 billion.

The preponderance of evidence on government forcing more money into the health system shows it does not increase preventive or primary

---

2008, page 20. Available at https://www.mahealthconnector.org/wp-content/uploads/annual-reports/ConnectorAnnualReport2008.pdf; "Report to the Massachusetts Legislature, Implementation of Health Care Reform, Fiscal Year 2013," Massachusetts Health Connector, January 2014, page 9. Available at https://www.mahealthconnector.org/wpcontent/uploads/annual-reports/ConnectorAnnualReport2013.pdf.

[9] Liz Kowalczyk, "ER visits, costs in Mass. Climb," Boston Globe, April 24, 2009. Available at http://archive.boston.com/news/local/massachusetts/articles/2009/04/24/er_visits_costs_in_mass_climb/.

[10] "Patrick-Murray Administration's Division of Insurance Announces Decision on Rate Increase Submissions by Health Insurers,' press release, Massachusetts Division of Insurance, April 1, 2010.

[11] Robert Weisman, "State Acts to Oversee 3 Insurers, Boston Globe, June 11, 2010.

[12] "Health Plan Choice and Premiums in the 2017 Health Insurance Marketplace," U.S. Department of Health & Human Services, October 24, 2016, page 5. Available at https://aspe.hhs.gov/sites/default/files/pdf/212721/2017MarketplaceLandscapeBrief.pdf.

[13] Thomas DeLeire, Karen Joynt, and Ruth McDonald, "Impact of Insurance Expansion on Hospital Uncompensated Care Costs," U.S. Department of Health & Human Services, September 24, 2014, page 1. Available at https://aspe.hhs.gov/pdf-report/impact-insurance-expansion-hospital-uncompensated-care-costs-2014.

care and reduce emergency department use. Plenty of evidence, reaching as far back as the Canadian province of Quebec's guaranteeing universal coverage in 1971 shows emergency departments see more patients, not fewer, after such a reform.[14]

What such reforms do achieve is to feed more unaccountable money into hospitals and other health services facilities. If we look back in a straight line from December 2016 to January 2008, the high-water mark of employment before the Great Recession started destroying jobs, we can see the United States added 6.87 million nonfarm civilian jobs. (This is the net figure, passing over the millions of jobs lost and re-gained through the recession). However, 2.59 million jobs are in health services, which grew by one fifth (20 percent). All other nonfarm jobs grew only 3.42 percent, adding 4.29 million jobs. Health services accounted for 38 percent of all jobs added from the January 2008 peak through the end of last year.[15]

The evidence shows an individual mandate to maintain health insurance is not an appropriate government measure to induce residents to take responsibility for their health. Rather, it gives cover for a dramatic increase in government spending on a health services sector that shows no productivity improvements.

Chairman BUCHANAN. Mr. Miller, you are up next.

STATEMENT OF THOMAS MILLER, RESIDENT FELLOW, AMERICAN ENTERPRISE INSTITUTE

Mr. MILLER. Thank you, Chairman Buchanan, Ranking Member Lewis, Members of the Subcommittee, for the opportunity to testify today

---

[14] John R. Graham, "Least Surprising Health Research Result Ever: Medicaid Increases ER Use," Health Policy Blog, National Center for Policy Analysis, January 16, 2014. Available at http://healthblog.ncpa.org/least-surprisinghealth-research-result-ever-medicaid-increases-er-use/#sthash.16xwCVES.ItBX25u8.dpbs.

[15] John R. Graham, "Obamacare's Voodoo Employment Economics Threatens Reform," National Center for Policy Analysis, forthcoming.

to examine the effectiveness of the individual mandate under the Affordable Care Act.

The shaky case for the individual mandate is based on mistaken premises, faulty economic analysis, shortsighted politics, and flawed health policy. Opponents have found the mandate to be administratively challenging, politically unsustainable, economically unnecessary, beyond the scope of a proper role of government, and constitutionally questionable.

Most arguments in favor of the individual mandate usually present it as a necessary, though far less popular, means to more laudable ends. Well, they certainly got the last part right. The individual mandate touches exposed nerves and offends core principles in ways that other elements of the modern regulatory state do not. The individual mandate has consistently remained the most intensely unpopular provision of the new health care law since it first took shape.

One of strongest driving forces behind officeholders resorting to the individual mandate is the desire to substitute off-budget mandated private funds in place of more visible taxes that they would otherwise find hard to impose to meet their insurance coverage goals and finance additional health care spending. But shifting costs less transparently is not the same as actually reducing them.

The type of mandate that the U.S. political economy and health care system is likely to deliver in practice is very different and more complicated than what might be assumed under best case theories. Trying to force people to buy insurance they cannot afford or pay much more for such coverage than it actually appears worth to them remains politically and economically difficult.

As a consequence, the individual mandate continues to face significant political limits on how large the mandate's penalties can be, how aggressively they can be enforced, and how much compliance the mandate will produce. Hence, the mandate's best future for continued survival involves operating much more as a gentle suggestion or nudge rather than a more polarizing command. Because the penalties for failing to comply with the mandate are rather modest in proportion to the average—likely average premium cost of required coverage, millions of individuals have calculated that it is much less expensive to pay the penalty than to purchase mandatory insurance.

Projections for compliance versus penalty payment under the individual mandate by the Congressional Budget Office consistently have overestimated the degree of compliance. In practice, the Internal Revenue Service has reported noticeably higher numbers of individual mandate penalty payers despite lower amounts of actual revenue collected. CBO also has tended to be on the high side of claims that the Affordable Care Act would rapidly and substantially increase coverage in the new law's exchanges for individual coverage as well.

Rather than reexamine the flawed foundations of its previous assumptions, CBO appears to have recently doubled down on them. The CBO estimates are flawed in overstating baseline assumptions for future growth in the ACA's version of individual market coverage, exaggerating the response rate of those subject to the mandate before and after its possible repeal, misestimating Medicaid coverage effects, and setting unrealistic parameters for future health policy changes. In fact, the most significant force behind the size and shape of insurance coverage gains has been large taxpayer subsidies primarily through the expanded Medicaid program.

Enrollment rates for the ACA exchanges are highly sensitive to one's income and premium tax subsidy level. Enrollment by younger and healthier risks, which is supposed to be the primary target of the individual mandate, has failed to reach expected levels. There are a variety of alternative policy remedies that could be pursued if the individual mandate is either limited further or repealed. They include extension of HIPAA-like protection against health status risk rating to individuals in the nongroup market who maintain continuous qualified insurance coverage while switching between health plans. Or imposing penalties in the form of higher insurance premium surcharges when eligible individuals fail to obtain or maintain minimum qualified coverage during annual open enrollment periods. Or tightening eligibility verification further for special enrollment periods between annual open seasons in ACA exchanges. Or enabling default enrollment in minimum qualified coverage costing no more than the value of applicable Federal taxpayer subsidies for insurance. Or providing a different mix of taxpayer subsidies for obtaining and maintaining qualified insurance coverage in the individual market that are more generous to younger and healthier individuals who have declined coverage thus far. Or as a last resort for some and a first resort for others, actually enabling and incentivizing insurers to offer coverage that is less expensive and more attractive to potential uninsured customers.

Thank you, Mr. Chairman. I look forward to your questions.

Chairman BUCHANAN. Thank you, Mr. Miller.

[The prepared statement of Mr. Miller follows:]

STATEMENT BEFORE THE HOUSE COMMITTEE ON WAYS AND MEANS SUBCOMMITTEE ON OVERSIGHT

Examining the Effectiveness of the Individual Mandate under the Affordable Care Act

Thomas P. Miller, J.D.
Resident Fellow in Health Policy Studies
January 24, 2017

Thank you Chairman Buchanan, Subcommittee Ranking Member Lewis, and Members of the Subcommittee for the opportunity to testify today to examine the effectiveness of the individual mandate under the Affordable Care Act (ACA).

I am testifying today as a health policy researcher and a resident fellow at the American Enterprise Institute (AEI). I also will draw upon previous experience as a senior health economist at the Joint Economic Committee and health policy researcher at several other Washington-based research organizations.

My testimony will outline the rationales and motivations behind use of the individual mandate within the ACA and then examine its disappointing record in trying to achieve its goals. I will summarize the inherent political, economic, and legal limits in attempting to implement and enforce a strong mandate, as well as the potential dangers and drawbacks in doing so. Finally, I will suggest that we need to distinguish the actual effects of the mandate from those due to other health policy changes, either in increasing insurance coverage or limiting its costs. I will conclude by outlining a variety of alternative policy remedies that could be pursued if the individual mandate is either weakened further or repealed.

The shaky case for the individual mandate is based on mistaken premises, faulty economic analysis, short-sighted politics, and flawed health policy. Opponents have found the mandate to be administratively challenging, politically unsustainable, economically unnecessary, beyond the proper role of government, and constitutionally questionable.

Arguments in favor of the individual mandate usually present it as a necessary, though far less popular, means to more laudable ends such as universal coverage, better access to health care for persons with preexisting health conditions, and lower health care costs for those already insured. However, the relationship between the mandate and the problems it purportedly could solve always has been tenuous and contradictory at best. It turns out that the type of mandate that the U.S. political economy and health care system is likely to deliver in practice is very different and more complicated than what might be assumed under best-case theories.

Rearranging Increased Coverage Costs

One of the strongest driving forces behind officeholders resorting to the individual mandate is the desire to substitute "off-budget" mandated private funds in place of more visible taxes that they would otherwise find hard to impose to meet their insurance coverage goals and finance additional health care spending. Making the full costs of mandatory coverage more transparent reduces popular support for the latter. The hope instead is that an individual mandate can obscure the full sticker-price shock to taxpayers because mandated private spending is not officially treated as part of the federal budget. Instead, employers and insurers are enlisted as surrogate "tax collectors" through less transparent and politically accountable means.

Not surprisingly an individual mandate has the least support from those it is purported to help: people who currently do not enroll in public coverage or employer-sponsored insurance or who do not already purchase individual-market coverage. After all, coercing some people to do what they otherwise would not is the very point of a legal mandate. However, trying to force them to buy insurance they cannot afford or pay more for such coverage than it actually appears to be worth to them remains politically difficult.

Hence, an individual mandate often promises, but never manages, to pay for itself. In order to get lower-income individuals to comply with a mandate to purchase more insurance than they can afford, or want to purchase, substantial taxpayer subsidies are used to fill some of the affordability gap. Insurance mandates create a perpetual conflict between their escalating costs, limited public and private resources to pay for them, and the false guarantees of richer coverage ahead. The imbalances may be financed through various combinations of higher taxes, reduced benefits, higher premiums, lower take-home pay, fewer economic opportunities, and less insurance coverage for everyone else. Doing so also reduces portions of any projected increases in new premium "revenue" expected by insurers and health care providers from expanded coverage. Eventually, some of those less-visible costs are reimposed on the initially more "fortunate" newly insured.

Weak Enforcement

In their comprehensive review of the likely efficacy of mandates for health insurance, Glied, Hartz, and Giorgi (2007) concluded that predicting a target population's response to a mandate is, at best, an inexact science. Performance of mandates varies greatly with such important factors as the affordability of costs of compliance, the size of penalties, and the probability that penalties will be imposed in a timely manner. Glied, Hartz, and Giorgi also noted that even the best mandate is unlikely to affect the behavior of those who are transient (in terms of place of residence or employment status) and have few assets.

Some modelers of the coverage take-up effects of an individual mandate appear to assume reflexively that its commands will be obeyed faithfully, enforced consistently, and executed with nearly flawless precision. Actual enforcement practice under the ACA provides more of a muffled bark and toothless bite.

One early indication was that the mandate did not even begin to apply until January 1, 2014, even though the law was enacted in March 2010. Although the mandate penalties were supposed to be enforced by the Internal Revenue Service and collected through taxpayers' annual income tax returns, the agency is not allowed to use many of its standard enforcement tools to ensure payment of those taxes. The law provides that anyone who fails to pay in a timely

manner any penalty imposed by the mandate "shall not be subject to any criminal prosecution or penalty" and that the secretary of the Treasury shall not "file notice of lien" or "levy" on any property of a taxpayer by reason of such failure.[16]

The penalties for failing to comply with the mandate also are rather modest in proportion to the likely average premium cost of required coverage.[17] The predictable result was that millions of individuals calculated that it is much less expensive to pay the penalty than to purchase mandatory insurance. The law's guaranteed-issue incentives for potential purchasers, coupled with loose enforcement of eligibility for special enrollment periods between annual open season windows, encouraged

---

[16] Patient Protection and Affordable Care Act, 2010, section 1501(g)(2)(A) and (B)(i-1)]).

[17] The penalty is the greater of a flat-dollar amount or a percentage of the violator's income. After the penalty amounts were phased in over three years (ending in 2016), the flat-dollar version equaled $695 per individual, and the percentage-of-income version equaled 2.5 percent of income. The total family penalty for the flat-dollar version is capped at 300% of the amount per individual. The total monthly penalty for a taxpayer and his or her dependents for the percentage-of-income version cannot be more than the cost of the national average premium for bronze-level health plans (60 percent actuarial value) offered through health insurance exchanges (for the relevant family size). The latter penalty amount can be multiplied by the number of individuals in a family subject to a penalty, up to a maximum of five individuals. The flat dollar penalty amount is indexed to increase at the rate of inflation in years after 2016.

individuals to enroll "just in time" when sick and "go bare" when healthy and pay less in penalties than in total premiums), further ensuring limited and erratic mandate compliance.

Moreover, the ACA provisions for exemptions from the individual mandate – involving illegal immigrants, foreign nationals, religious prohibitions, and most importantly "unaffordability"[18] in all reveal how various political and economic factors limit the enforceable scope of any theoretically universal mandate. Once the individual mandate was first put into effect for the 2014 plan year, other permissive exemptions were added, for such excuses as recent death of a close family member, facing evictions, and having medical expenses that could not be paid in the last 24 months that resulted in substantial debt. In addition, reliance on the federal income tax system and the IRS as primary enforcers of the mandate fails to reach millions of Americans who are not required to (or do not) file a federal income tax return. The penalty is pro-rated for people who are uninsured for a portion of the year and waived for people who have a period without insurance of less than three months.

Ironically, even the strongest version of an individual mandate to purchase health insurance would be too weak to guarantee what should be its ultimate objective – improvements in people's health. Requiring that someone have health insurance is not the same as ensuring they actually receive all of the effective health care services they may need in a timely manner and comply with their physicians' advice, let alone that we all take many other steps beyond even the delivery of covered medical services that might do more to improve their current and future health. To do that, one might need to mandate not just the purchase of health insurance but also delivery of the actual treatment"! Yet somehow the image of a mandate that all preventive and therapeutic treatment" be received at the right time and right place (or even the right physical point of entry?) with no questions asked or informed consent required suggests more vividly the limits of government coercion in achieving health goals.

---

[18] Unaffordability in the ACA statute is defined as when one's required health premium costs would be greater than 8 percent of household income, beginning in 2014. This unaffordability measure has been subsequently indexed upward to 8.13 percent for 2016.

Weak Compliance

Projections for compliance versus penalty payment under the individual mandate by the Congressional Budget Office (CBO) have tended to overestimate the degree of compliance, but in a choppy manner. For example, using 2016 as a baseline year, CBO first projected in April 2010 that the ACA's individual mandate would help produce more coverage of the uninsured and collect only $4.2 billion in mandate penalties from 3.9 million individuals, even while leaving 13-14 million Americans exempt from its reach. In 2012, CBO revised those numbers to project a higher amount of $6.9 billion in mandate penalties from about 5.9 million individuals. In 2014, CBO lowered those estimates to $4.2 billion, to be collected from about 3.9 million individuals. In 2016, the CBO estimates dipped slightly again, to $3 billion collected from a monthly average of 3 million individuals. CBO's reported estimates regarding the number of exempted individuals for the years 2014-2016 are not reported in a consistent manner, particularly in distinguishing between individuals who did not have to report on compliance because they were exempt from filing federal income taxes and others who were exempt from the individual mandate for other reasons.

These varying estimates somewhat reflect changes in underlying assumptions, reporting methods, and ACA implementation policy, but they also suggest their inexact nature and limited degrees of predictive accuracy. In practice, the IRS has reported noticeably higher numbers of individual mandate penalty payers (7.5 million in 2014, 6.5 million in 2015), despite lower amounts of actual revenue collected ($1.5 billion in 2014, $1.7 billion in 2015). The IRS also reports that about 12 million individuals in 2014 and 12.7 million individuals in 2015 were exempted from the mandate. (The 2015 estimates are preliminary and likely to grow somewhat higher, based on past trends).

Still the Most Unpopular Part of the ACA

The individual mandate issues touches expose nerves and offends core principles in ways that other elements of the modern regulatory state do not. Many Americans remain troubled by the idea of Congress imposing a legal mandate on citizens to purchase a private (but highly regulated) product, regardless of their wishes. They worry that implementing an individual mandate inevitably generates more and more rules regarding exactly what it requires, how it is carried out, and who pays for it. Hence, the individual mandate has consistently remained the most intensely unpopular provision of the new health law since it first took shape. For example, the November Kaiser Health Tracking Poll conducted shortly after the November elections found that only 35 percent of all Americans held favorable views about the individual mandate.[19]

Concerns that an individual mandate violates basic principles of economic freedom, personal choice, and limited government under the U.S. Constitution have persisted years after the Sunreme Court's narrowly divided decision in *NFIB v. Sebelius* to unhold the ACA mandate as a constitutionally valid exercise of the congressional power to tax, rather than as a regulatory penalty under the power of Congress to regulate interstate commerce.[20] It appears that the individual mandate remains politically unpopular whether it is viewed as a limited regulatory penalty to spur more purchasing of required health insurance or a modest tax to help finance subsidies to do so.

Reciprocal Floors and Ceilings Limit the Individual Mandate

The ACA's individual mandate was primarily designed to help fill in the gaps between what the law's advocates could deliver politically in larger taxpayer subsidies for expanded health insurance coverage and the higher costs of coverage produced by more aggressive regulation of health

---

[19] Ashley Kirzinger, Elise Sugarman, and Mollyann Brodie, Kaiser Health Tracking Poll: November 2016, Kaiser Family Foundation, December 1, 2016, Figure 11, http://kfl.org health-costs poll-finding kaiser-health-tracking. poll-november 2016. See also Dennis Thompson, "6 Years Later, Obamacare Still Divides America: Poll." HealthDay, May 5, 2016. (Table 3 notes a Harris Poll finding that 64 percent of U.S. adults would like to repeal the ACA's individual mandate), http://www.theharrispoll.com/polities/Obamacare-Still-Divides-America html.

[20] See Thomas A. Lambert, "How the Supreme Court Doomed the ACA to Failure," Regulation, Winter 2012-2013, https://object.cato.org/sites/cato.org/files/serials/files/regulation/2013/1/v35n4-5.pdf, asserting that Chief Justice Roberts' majority opinion also means that the penalty for failure to carry health insurance can count as a tax for irposes, and remain a valid exercise of congressional power, but only if it is kept so small as to be largely ineffective.

insurance. It essentially aimed to require less-cost, low-risk individuals not only to obtain or retain federally-mandated minimum essential coverage, but also to pay more for it, in order to cross-subsidize lower premiums for other high-risk and/or low-income individuals. However, the individual mandate continues to face significant political limits on how large the mandate's penalties can be, how aggressively they can be enforced, and how much compliance the mandate will produce. Hence, the mandate's best future for continued survival involves operating much more as a gentle "suggestion" or nudge (with modest penalties and weak enforcement) rather than a more polarizing "command."

In short, the space separating the floor and ceiling for the individual mandate is narrow. If the individual mandate ever begins the reach the point in practice at which it threatens to become more binding and effective, political feedback and pressure to pull back will intensify.

Impact on Insurance Coverage Expansion?

It's a fact that health insurance coverage has increased significantly since the ACA was enacted into law and implemented. The causal factors are more complex and contestable.

CBO has tended to be on the high side of claims that the ACA would rapidly and substantially increase coverage in the new law's exchanges (later renamed "Marketplaces") for individual coverage. It also has repeatedly overestimated the role of the individual mandate in delivering such gains. CBO's original projections assumed far more stability in the exchanges by now, and much larger enrollment in them (about 21-22 million people, rather than a little more than half that number). Rather than reexamine the flawed foundations of its previous assumptions, CBO appears to have recently doubled down on them in projecting that a partial repeal of the ACA (similar to one passed by Congress but vetoed in January 2016), without additional provisions to replace it, would increase the number of uninsured by 18 million in 2018, 27 million in 2020, and 32 million in 2026.

The CBO estimates are flawed in overstating its baseline assumptions for future growth in the ACA's version of individual market coverage, exaggerating the response rate of those subject to the individual mandate before and after its possible repeal, misestimating Medicaid coverage effects, and setting unrealistic parameters for future health policy changes.[21]

To be fair, the ACA in practice has evolved through numerous iterations of interrelated moving parts, unforeseen modifications in policies and practices, and changes in economic assumptions. However, it's still accurate to conclude that the most significant force behind the size and shape of insurance coverage gains has been large taxpayer subsidies, particularly through the expanded Medicaid program. Indeed, even the most recent estimate by one of the ACA's past architects, Jonathan Gruber, concluded that overall coverage rates in 2014 did not respond to either the mandate's penalties or exemptions for lacking coverage. Gruber and his co authors did find that Medicaid accounted for 63 percent of the coverage gains in 2014 that their methods could identify, and that the fairly modest effects of the law's premium subsidies for ACA exchange coverage accounted for the rest.[22]

This type of analysis is consistent with other findings that enrollment rates for ACA exchanges are sensitive to one's income and premium tax credit subsidy level,[23] and that enrollment by younger and healthier risks -

---

[21] See, e.g., Brian Blasé, "Learning from CBO's History of Incorrect ObamaCare Projections." The Apothecary, January 2, 2017. http://www.forbes.com/sites/theapothecary/2017-01-02/learning-from-cbos-history-of-incorrectobamacare-projections print: Avik Roy, "Four Critical Problems with the CBO's Latest Obamacare Repeal Estimates, The Apothecary, January 17, 2017, http://www.forbes.com/sites/theapothecary/2017/01/17/four-criticalproblems-with-the-cbos-latest-obamacare-repeal-estimates/#1292a6b77862.

[22] Molly Frean, Jonathan Gruber, and Benjamin D. Sommers, "Disentangling the ACA's Coverage Effects Lessons for Policymakers," New England Journal of Medicine, 375, no. 17 (2016): 1605-1607. See also Molly Frean, Jonathan Gruber, and Benjamin D. Sommers, "Premium Subsidies, the Mandate, and Medicaid Expansion: Coverage Effects of the Affordable Care Act, National Bureau of Economic Research Working Paper no. 22213 April 2016 (finding that the mandate penalty had a negligible impact on coverage").

[23] Caroline F. Pearson, "Exchanges Struggle to Enroll Consumers as Income Increases," Avalere, March 25, 2015, http://avalere.com/expertise/managed-care/insights/exchanges-struggle-to-enroll-consumers-as-incomeincreases.

the primary targets of the individual mandate – has failed to reach expected levels.[24]

Future Unknowns

Given that the practical consequences of the individual mandate in increasing insurance market coverage appear to be minimal, at best, what accounts for other sources of support or opposition to it? One well-worn hope is that the individual mandate can help to strengthen and lock in the effects of other ACA health insurance regulations for minimum essential health benefits, qualified health plans, adjusted community rating, and guaranteed issue, in part by reducing their most visible on-budget costs. The ultimate aim on the regulatory side would be to make the purchase of any other alternative health care arrangements all but impossible.

Opponents of the individual mandate want to short-circuit any future evolution of a stronger mandate that requires compliance with potentially more sweeping regulations not yet implemented, or even proposed. Hence, a large portion of the ongoing debate over the individual mandate is as much about what it might become later than what it is currently.

Alternatives

Focus on the individual mandate in the ACA's drafting, implementation, and post enactment debate has tended to obscure and preempt consideration of other policy alternatives.

They include:

- Extension of HIPAA-like protection against health status risk-rating to individuals who maintain "continuous" qualified insurance coverage while switching between individual market health plans or between group-market and individual-market plans,
- Imposing penalties in the form of higher insurance premium surcharges for each time that an individual fails to obtain or

---

[24] Brian Blasé, "Obamacare's Failure and Moving Health Care Policy in a New Direction, The Apothecary, December 15, 2016, http://wwwforbes.com/sites/theapothecary/2016/12/15/obamcares-failure-and-moving-healthcare-policy-in-a-new-direction/print/.

maintain minimum qualified coverage during annual open enrollment periods. This would operate somewhat like the delayed enrollment penalty for coverage in Medicare Part B or Medicare Part D.[25]

- Tightening eligibility and enforcement further for "special enrollment periods between annual open seasons in ACA exchanges
- Default enrollment in minimum qualified coverage costing no more than the value of applicable federal taxpayer subsidies for insurance, provided that sufficient notice and simple mechanisms to "opt out" are ensured,
- Providing even more generous, but also more transparent, taxpayer subsidies for obtaining and maintaining qualified insurance coverage in the individual market. This would emulate part of the success of employer-sponsored insurance and federal employee health benefits program coverage, albeit at an even-higher per-enrollee budgetary cost.
- Enabling and incentivizing insurers to offer coverage that is less expensive and more attractive to potential uninsured customers.

Of course, the last option --- though closest to market-based, competitive, patientcentered health insurance -- is likely to be considered only as a last resort if and when the other policy options fail!

Chairman BUCHANAN. Dr. McDonough, it is your testimony.

---

[25] The penalty would not necessarily be cumulative over one's remaining lifetime if one "requalifies" again by obtaining and maintaining such coverage in several subsequent, consecutive years.

STATEMENT OF JOHN E. MCDONOUGH, DRPH, MPA, PROFESSOR OF PRACTICE, DEPARTMENT OF HEALTH POLICY AND MANAGEMENT, HARVARD TH CHAN SCHOOL OF PUBLIC HEALTH

Mr. MCDONOUGH. Thank you, Chairman Buchanan and Ranking Member Lewis and Members of the Committee.

Chairman BUCHANAN. Turn your mike on.

Mr. MCDONOUGH. Pardon me. Thank you.

Thank you, Chairman Buchanan, Ranking Member Lewis, Members of the Committee. I am John McDonough from the Harvard Chan School of Public Health. I would just note from my bio in my statement that I, between 2008 and 2010, was a staff person for the Senate Committee on Health, Education, Labor, and Pensions, and worked on the writing and passage of the Affordable Care Act. So I am a former Senate staff person in recovery. And I think most of you will understand that that is unfortunately a terminal, lifelong preexisting condition that I just can't shake as much as I might try.

So thank you for the honor of speaking before you. I have a written statement, and I will just highlight my six main points in it and then engage in conversation on whatever matters you find of value talking with me about.

First, the individual mandate, so-called the individual responsibility requirement of the ACA, is a core mechanism to ensure a healthy risk pool and more stable premiums in a guaranteed issue market that bans the practice of medical underwriting and preexisting condition exclusions in the individual health insurance market. It is core and it is recognized, and is not the only way to address it, but it is an essential component of the law. What we in Massachusetts where I was involved in the passage of the Massachusetts health reform law refer to as the three-legged stool.

Secondly, to eliminate the mandate and to leave in place guaranteed issue is a sure and proven formula for major disruption in the individual health insurance market nationally. And that is a concern that I think is neither speculative nor hypothetical. We have seen it played out in a number of States over the past 25 years.

Thirdly, I would mention, as Dr. Graham has also mentioned, that between the late 1980s and the latter part of the last decade, the individual mandate was largely a policy idea that was championed by conservatives, starting with Professor Mark Pauly and Stuart Butler in the late 1980s. And only in the latter part of the last decade was it embraced and accepted by Democrats. Its roots are entirely based on the notion of individual responsibility and shared responsibility as Governor Mitt Romney stated repeatedly during the Massachusetts health reform experience.

Fourthly, there are other ways to get at the intent and purpose of the individual mandate. It is not that mechanism or anything else. One mechanism is in late enrollment penalties. Another mechanism is referenced in Speaker Ryan's Better Way plan in terms of continuous coverage requirements. I would caution that I think that if you compare the individual mandate and continuous coverage requirements, I would regard the continuous coverage requirements as far more onerous and punitive in terms of consumers and would urge caution before you go too far down that path.

Fifthly, I find no empirical evidence that suggests that the individual mandate has anything to do with the stresses that have been experienced in the State and Federal health insurance exchanges over the 2007 enrollment and now carrying-out period. There are other causes that I think more effectively explain those problems that are going on in those markets and be happy to talk with you about those.

And finally, I would only suggest that the suggestion that the size of the individual mandate penalty should be increased to enhance the uptake of individual health insurance is a mistaken notion. I think far more at the core in terms of enhancing enrollment would be to address the lack of adequate affordability in the health insurance exchanges right now, particularly for consumers between 250 and 400 percent of the Federal poverty level.

Those are my main points, and I look forward to further conversation. Thank you.

Chairman BUCHANAN. Thank you, Doctor.

[The prepared statement of Dr. John E McDonough, DrPH, MPA follows:]

Comments for the Record U.S. House Committee on Ways and Means, Subcommittee on Oversight Hearing on Health Insurance Individual Responsibility

Tuesday, January 24, 2017
By Dr. John E. McDonough
Harvard TH Chan School of Public Health

Chairman Buchanan, Ranking Member Lewis, and members of the Subcommittee on Oversight, my name is John E McDonough and I am a professor of practice in the Department of Health Policy and Management at the Harvard T.H. Chan School of Public Health in Boston, Massachusetts. I hold a doctoral degree in public health and a master's degree in public administration. Formerly I worked between 2008 and 2010 as a senior advisor on national health reform for the U.S. Senate Committee on Health, Education, Labor and Pensions where I participated in the writing and passage of the Affordable Care Act (ACA). Between 2003 and 2008, I served as executive director of Health Care for All, Massachusetts' leading consumer health advocacy organization where I was deeply involved in the passage and implementation of the 2006 Massachusetts Health Reform Law. Between 1985 and 1997, I served as a member of the Massachusetts House of Representatives where I held many health policy positions of responsibility, including co-chair of the committees on health care and insurance.

I am here to offer testimony on the ACA's "requirement to maintain minimum essential coverage" (Section 1501, 42 USC 18091), as well as a similar provision enacted as part of the 2006 Massachusetts health reform law that served as a model for Title 1 of the ACA. Though popularly -- or unpopularly-known as the "individual mandate," that term is not used in either federal or state statutes to describe the "individual responsibility provisions of the law. I advance six points, outlined below:

during the 1990s. When the damage from guaranteed issue without some form of mandate became evident, some states abandoned the protections, while other states accepted the damage to their individual market risk pool and continued the practice.

As of 2012, only five states (Maine, Massachusetts, New Jersey, New York, and Vermont) required individual market health insurers to guarantee issue all products to all residents. These five states maintained their guaranteed issue requirements despite a collapse in participation by individual consumers in the face of growing unaffordable health insurance premiums. The impact was most dramatically evident in New York State where participation in the individual market dropped from 752,000 covered lives in the early 1990s when guaranteed issue was first adopted to about 34,000 covered lives in 2009.[31] Massachusetts saw a similar form of insurance "death spiral" when it adopted guaranteed issue in its individual health insurance market in 1996 without an accompanying mandate, only seeing the non-group market return to viability after implementation of the state's individual mandate in 2007.[32] Other states, notably New Hampshire, Kentucky, and Washington repealed or restricted their guaranteed issue rules once the market impact became clear. Four states (Michigan, Pennsylvania, Rhode Island, and Virginia, plus the District of Columbia) in 2012 still required their Blue Cross Blue Shield carrier to act as insurer of last resort, an increasingly unworkable formula as the cost of care for clients in the individual markets became increasingly unsustainable.[33]

Though guaranteed issue and the related banning of medical underwriting and pre-existing condition exclusions remain among the most popular features of the ACA, with public promises to retain it from President Trump, House Speaker Ryan, and Senate Majority Leader

---

[31] G. C. Sandler. "New York Individual Market Rules: The Nuts and Bolts of Rating in the Individual Market." National Health Policy Forum, Washington DC, February 19, 2009, slide 4.
[32] M. Hackmann et al. "Adverse Selection and an Individual Mandate: When Theory Meets Practice." American Economic Review. 2015 Mar; 105(3): 1030-66. Available at: https://www.ncbi.nlm.nih.gov/pmc/articles/PMC4408001/ (accessed 1-20-2017).
[33] Kaiser Family Foundation. "Health Insurance Market Reforms: Guaranteed Issue." Focus on Health Reform. June 2012. Available at: https://kaiserfamilyfoundation.files.wordpress.com/2013/01/8327.pdf (accessed 1-18-2017).

- The individual mandate is a core mechanism to ensure a healthy risk pool and more stable premiums in a guaranteed issue market that bans the practices of medical underwriting and pre-existing condition exclusions in insurance contracting in the individual market.
- To eliminate the mandate and leave in place guaranteed issue is a sure and proven formula for major disruption in the individual health insurance market nationally, a concern that is neither speculative nor hypothetical.
- Between the late 1980s and 2009, the individual mandate was largely an idea championed by both conservative and moderate Republicans until former President Barack Obama endorsed it in June 2009.
- Other mechanisms could be used to replace the individual mandate, such as late enrollment penalties or the proposed "continuous coverage" requirement advanced in Speaker Paul Ryan's "Better Way" health proposal, though the latter requirement would be far more punitive towards individual consumers than the ACA's individual mandate.
- No empirical evidence I can find suggests that the individual mandate is the cause of the stresses recently experienced during the 2017 enrollment cycle in many of the federal and state health insurance exchanges. Other causes more effectively explain these recent problems.
- Finally, the suggestion that the size of the individual mandate's tax penalty should be increased to enhance the uptake of individual health insurance is misguided. More effective would be increasing premium and cost sharing subsidies for income eligible consumers to more closely mirror affordability levels in the Massachusetts health insurance system.

I will elaborate on these in turn.

First, the individual mandate is a core mechanism to ensure a healthy risk pool and more stable premiums in a guaranteed issue market that bans

the practices of medical underwriting and pre-existing condition exclusions in insurance contracting in the individual market.

In the 2006 Massachusetts and 2010 U.S. health reform laws, the individual mandate was recognized as an essential component of a "three-legged stool" to expand health insurance coverage, especially in the private individual (non-group) health insurance market. The other two legs are: first, guaranteed issue of individual health insurance to all qualified persons regardless of medical history or current health status; and second, premium and cost sharing support/subsidies to make the purchase of health insurance affordable for those who would otherwise be unable to afford the cost of coverage. Like a stool, all three of the legs are necessary for the structure to stand reliably.

The "three-legged stool" structure, including the individual mandate, has proven effective in the achievement of a principal goal of both the Massachusetts and U.S. health reform laws, that is the lowering of the numbers of persons without insurance. In Massachusetts, the rate of uninsured dropped from 7.7% in 2006 to 2.5% in 2015.[26] In the U.S. the number of uninsured Americans has dropped from 48.6 million in 2010 to 28.6 million in 2015.[27] The U.S. uninsurance rate, now between 8-9%, is the lowest it has even been recorded in the nation.

Research studies have reached differing conclusions on the precise impact of the individual mandate itself in achieving these reductions in rates and numbers of uninsured. For example, in a 2015 RAND Research Brief, Eibner and Saltzman found that the absence of the ACA mandate would lead to a 20% drop in individual market enrollment, and a 27% drop in enrollment among young adults.[28] On the other hand, Frean et al in a 2016 Working Paper for the National Bureau of Economic Research, found only "small and inconsistent effects of the individual mandate in 2014 and 2015 with minimal policy impact."[29]

Regardless of the empirical evidence, the health insurance industry as well as health insurance experts have been clear for nearly three decades that some form of a coverage obligation is essential to provide a balanced risk pool and to provide necessary confidence that guaranteed issue can be maintained in a financially sustainable manner. A December 7 2016 letter to Speaker Paul Ryan and Leader Nancy Pelosi from the American Academy of Actuaries describes this dynamic well:

> "A sustainable health insurance market depends on enrolling enough healthy people over which the costs of the less healthy people can be spread. To ensure viability when there is a guarantee that consumers with pre-existing conditions can obtain health insurance coverage at standard rates requires mechanisms to spread the cost of that guarantee over a broad population. The ACA's individual mandate encourages even the young and healthy to obtain coverage."[30]

Among health insurance and health policy experts, widespread consensus exists that to maintain guaranteed issue without any pre-existing condition exclusions requires some enforceable mechanism to provide a robust and diverse risk profile among eligible consumers.

Second, to eliminate the mandate and leave in place guaranteed issue is a sure and proven formula for major disruption in the individual health insurance market nationally, a concern that is neither speculative nor hypothetical.

The experiences of states between the early 1990s and today demonstrates that the concern about the workability of guaranteed issue without some enforceable mechanism such as an individual mandate is a legitimate and essential issue. Eight states adopted guaranteed issue, most

---

[26] S. Long et al. "Massachusetts Health Reform at Ten Years: Great Progress, But Coverage Gaps Remain." Health Affairs. 35, No. 9 (2016): 1633-1637. Available at: http://content.healthaffairs.org/content/35/9/1633.full.pdf+html (accessed 1-18-2017).

[27] B. Ward et al. "Early Release of Selected Estimates Based on Data from the 2015 National Health Interview Survey." National Center for Health Statistics, U.S. Centers for Disease Control and Prevention. May, 2016. Available at: https://www.cdc.gov/nchs/data/nhis/earlyrelease/earlyrelease201605.pdf (accessed 1-182016).

[28] Eibner C, Saltzman (2015). How does the ACA individual mandate affect enrollment and premiums in the individual insurance market? RAND Research Brief. Available at: http://www.rand.org/pubs/research_briefs/RB981224.html (accessed 1-16-17).

[29] Frean M, Gruber J, Sommers BD (2016). Premium subsidies, the mandate and Medicaid expansion: coverage effects of the Affordable Care Act. NBER Working Paper 22213. Available at http://www.nber.org/papers/w22213.pdf (accessed 1-17-2017).

[30] Shari Westerfield. Letter from American Academy of Actuaries to Speaker Paul Ryan and Leader Nancy Pelosi. December 7 2016. Available at: http://actuary.org/files/publications/HPC_letter_ACA_CSR_120716.pdf (accessed 1-18-17).

McConnell, the certain danger of maintaining guaranteed issue without an enforceable mandate of some form is neither speculative nor hypothetical. The Congressional Budget Office released a report as recently as January 17 concluding that "eliminating the mandate penalties and the subsidies while retaining the market reforms would destabilize the nongroup market and the effect would worsen over time."[34]

Third, between the late 1980s and 2009, the individual mandate was largely an idea championed by both conservative and moderate Republicans until former President Barack Obama endorsed it in June 2009.

The policy idea of a mandate on individuals to purchase health insurance as a mechanism to achieve near-universal coverage was introduced in the American health policy sphere in the late 1980s by Professor Mark Pauly of the University of Pennsylvania's Wharton School as an alternative to single-payer or employer mandate proposals to reach the same goal.[35] The idea was advanced and promoted by the Heritage Foundation, and especially by Dr. Stuart Butler, in the same period.[36] In the years 1993-1994 when the President Bill Clinton promoted national health reform legislation, Senators Robert Dole, John Chafee and Charles Grassley, along with 19 other Republican members of Congress as co-sponsors, advanced a proposal to establish a national mandate on most Americans to purchase health insurance as an alternative to the Clinton Administration's approach.[37] In the late 1990s, Louisiana Senator John Breaux became the first prominent Democrat to embrace the concept of the individual mandate.

---

[34] Congressional Budget Office. "How Repealing Portions of the Affordable Care Act Would Affect Health Insurance Coverage and Premiums." January 2017. Available at https://www.cbo.gov/sites/default/files/115th-congress2017-2018/reports/52371coverage andpremiums.pdf (accessed 1-18-2017).

[35] Pauly MV, Danzon P, Feldstein P and Hoff J (1991). A plan for 'responsible national health insurance.' Health Affairs 10(1): 5-25.

[36] Butler SM (1989). Assuring affordable health care for all Americans. Heritage Foundation. Accessed electronically 1/16/17 at http://www.heritage.org/research/lecture/assuring affordable-health-care-for-all-americans.

[37] M. Cooper. "Conservatives Sowed Idea of Health Care Mandate, Only to Spurn It Later." New York Time. February 14, 2012. Available at: http://www.nytimes.com/2012/02/15/ health/policy/health-care-mandate-was-first-backed-byconservatives.html (accessed 1-18-2017).

In 2004, Massachusetts Governor Mitt Romney proposed legislation to establish a statewide individual mandate that drew support from overwhelming Democratic majorities in the State Senate and House of Representatives, from U.S. Senator Edward Kennedy, and from President George W. Bush whose Administration provided key financing for the program. The legislation was signed into law on April 12, 2006 in a ceremony in Boston's historic Faneuil Hall. Seated on the stage was a representative of the Heritage Foundation which consulted with Governor Romney on structuring the individual mandate and creating the Massachusetts Health Insurance Connector Authority, the first governmental example of a health insurance exchange, another concept championed by the Heritage Foundation.[38]

The Massachusetts law incorporated the "three-legged stool" concept that is the organizing idea behind Title 1 of the ACA: systemic insurance market reform including guaranteed issue, an individual mandate to purchase health insurance, and premium/cost sharing subsidies to make the buying of insurance affordable. When Governor Romney left his position in January 2007 to begin his first campaign for the Republican nomination for U.S. President, full implementation of the law was left to his successor, Gov. Deval Patrick. During Romney's 2008 campaign, he received the endorsement of Sen. James De Mint who noted in his letter of support that as Governor, Romney had "passed innovative health care reforms."[39]

During the 2008 campaign for the Democratic nomination for U.S. President, leading candidates Hillary Clinton and John Edwards both advanced health care reform proposals that included an individual mandate, while candidate Barack Obama did not. Indeed, President Obama did not officially endorse inclusion of an individual mandate in health reform legislation until June 2009, well after the Congressional process had started in earnest. It was in this period that many Congressional Republicans began to distance themselves from the individual mandate.

---

[38] P. Belluck and K. Zezima. "Massachusetts Legislation on Insurance Becomes Law." New York Times. Available at: http://www.nytimes.com/2006/04/13/us/13health.html (accessed 1-18-2017).

[39] H. Hewitt. "Senator Jim DeMint Endorses Romney." Available at: http://www.hughhewitt.com/senator-jim-demint-endorses-romney-he-is-strongly-pro-life/ (accessed 1-18-2016).

Exemplifying this change was Senator Charles Grassley who stated on Fox News in June 2009: "When it comes to states requiring it for automobile insurance, the principle then ought to lie the same way for health insurance because everybody has some health insurance costs, and if you aren't insured, there's no free lunch. Somebody else is paying for it."[40] Three months later, in September 2009, his views had shifted: "Individuals should maintain the freedom to choose whether to purchase health insurance coverage or not.[41]

Democrats embraced the individual mandate concept in the 2000s in good faith to find common ground on universal coverage with Republicans and conservatives on a key structural feature championed by the latter groups. But as the ground shifted for Democrats leading them to support the mandate was a practical way forward, the ground shifted for Republicans compelling them to abandon a policy they had themselves promoted for nearly two decades.

Fourth, other mechanisms could be used to replace the individual mandate, such as late enrollment penalties or the proposed "continuous coverage" requirement advanced in Speaker Paul Ryan's "Better Way" health proposal, though the latter requirement would be more punitive towards individual consumers than the ACA's individual mandate.

Several mechanisms have been proposed to replace the ACA's individual mandate in replacement legislation. One of these is a "late penalty" fee such as the ones included in Medicare Parts B and D.[42] The alternative most often advanced in recent months is the proposal that guaranteed issue only be applied to individuals who maintain "continuous coverage" of their health insurance policies within defined limits. This proposal received prominent backing in the House Republican

---

[40] Transcript: Sens. Dodd, Grassley on FNS. Fox News Sunday, June 14 2009. Available at: http://www.foxnews.com/story/2009/06/14/transcript-sens-dodd-grassley-on-fns.html (accessed 1-18-17).
[41] Live Pulse. "Grassley Backtracks on Individual Mandate." Politico. September 22 2009. Available at: http://www.politico.com/livepulse/0909/Grassley backtracks on individual mandate.html (accessed 1-18-2017).
[42] J. Holahan and L. Blumberg. "Instead of ACA Repeal and Replace, Fix it." Urban Institute. January 2017. Available at: http://www.urban.org/research/publication/instead-aca-repealand-replace-fix-it/view/fullreport (accessed 1-20-2017).

Leadership's "A Better Way" health proposals released this past June 2016:

> "Our plan also proposes a new patient protection for those Americans who maintain continuous coverage. ... If an individual experiences a qualifying life event, he or she would not be charged more than standard rates - even if he or she is dealing with a serious medical issue. ... However, making the decision to forego coverage during this one-time open enrollment period will result in the forfeiture of continuous coverage protections and lead to higher health insurance coverage costs for that individual for a period in the future."[43]

Individuals and families unable to avoid undefined coverage gaps permitted under the Better Way plan would be subject to medical underwriting and pre-existing condition exclusions for, as mentioned above, "a period in the future." Those individuals with any pre-existing conditions found to relevant by health insurance companies for underwriting purposes would be denied coverage. Under the Better Way plan, their recourse for denied insurance applicants would be to seek coverage from newly re-established state high risk pools. The experience with state high risk pools has been mixed at best. Pools first established in the 1970s were chronically underfunded, often with long waiting lists and high premiums, with coverage limits that were banned by the ACA, such as lifetime and annual benefit caps, waiting periods, and limited benefits.[44]

Beyond these concerns is the issue of just how many individuals would be newly subjected to what I refer to as the "medical underwriting circle of hell." The current estimate of uninsured Americans by the CDC is 29 million, while the CBO estimates that as many as 32 million Americans potentially losing their insurance under Republican repeal legislation vetoed by President Obama one year ago. While we can hope that any

---

[43] House of Representatives. "A Better Way: Our Vision for a Confidant America." June 2016. Available at: http://abetterway.speaker.gov/_assets/pdf/ABetterWay-HealthCarePolicy Paper.pdf (accessed 1-18-2017).

[44] K. Pollitz. "High Risk Pools for Uninsurable Individuals." Kaiser Family Foundation. August 1, 2016. Available at: http://kff.org/health-reform/issue-brief/high-risk-pools-for-uninsurableindividuals/ (accessed 1-18-2017).

- The individual mandate is a core mechanism to ensure a healthy risk pool and more stable premiums in a guaranteed issue market that bans the practices of medical underwriting and pre-existing condition exclusions in insurance contracting in the individual market.
- To eliminate the mandate and leave in place guaranteed issue is a sure and proven formula for major disruption in the individual health insurance market nationally, a concern that is neither speculative nor hypothetical.
- Between the late 1980s and 2009, the individual mandate was largely an idea championed by both conservative and moderate Republicans until former President Barack Obama endorsed it in June 2009.
- Other mechanisms could be used to replace the individual mandate, such as late enrollment penalties or the proposed "continuous coverage" requirement advanced in Speaker Paul Ryan's "Better Way" health proposal, though the latter requirement would be far more punitive towards individual consumers than the ACA's individual mandate.
- No empirical evidence I can find suggests that the individual mandate is the cause of the stresses recently experienced during the 2017 enrollment cycle in many of the federal and state health insurance exchanges. Other causes more effectively explain these recent problems.
- Finally, the suggestion that the size of the individual mandate's tax penalty should be increased to enhance the uptake of individual health insurance is misguided. More effective would be increasing premium and cost sharing subsidies for income eligible consumers to more closely mirror affordability levels in the Massachusetts health insurance system.

I will elaborate on these in turn.

First, the individual mandate is a core mechanism to ensure a healthy risk pool and more stable premiums in a guaranteed issue market that bans the practices of medical underwriting and pre-existing condition exclusions in insurance contracting in the individual market.

In the 2006 Massachusetts and 2010 U.S. health reform laws, the individual mandate was recognized as an essential component of a "three-legged stool" to expand health insurance coverage, especially in the private individual (non-group) health insurance market. The other two legs are: first, guaranteed issue of individual health insurance to all qualified persons regardless of medical history or current health status; and second, premium and cost sharing support/subsidies to make the purchase of health insurance affordable for those who would otherwise be unable to afford the cost of coverage. Like a stool, all three of the legs are necessary for the structure to stand reliably.

The "three-legged stool" structure, including the individual mandate, has proven effective in the achievement of a principal goal of both the Massachusetts and U.S. health reform laws, that is the lowering of the numbers of persons without insurance. In Massachusetts, the rate of uninsured dropped from 7.7% in 2006 to 2.5% in 2015.[26] In the U.S. the number of uninsured Americans has dropped from 48.6 million in 2010 to 28.6 million in 2015.[27] The U.S. uninsurance rate, now between 8-9%, is the lowest it has even been recorded in the nation.

Research studies have reached differing conclusions on the precise impact of the individual mandate itself in achieving these reductions in rates and numbers of uninsured. For example, in a 2015 RAND Research Brief, Eibner and Saltzman found that the absence of the ACA mandate would lead to a 20% drop in individual market enrollment, and a 27% drop in enrollment among young adults.[28] On the other hand, Frean et al in a 2016 Working Paper for the National Bureau of Economic Research, found

---

[26] S. Long et al. "Massachusetts Health Reform at Ten Years: Great Progress, But Coverage Gaps Remain." Health Affairs. 35, No. 9 (2016): 1633-1637. Available at: http://content.healthaffairs.org/content/35/9/1633.full.pdf+html (accessed 1-18-2017).

[27] B. Ward et al. "Early Release of Selected Estimates Based on Data from the 2015 National Health Interview Survey." National Center for Health Statistics, U.S. Centers for Disease Control and Prevention. May, 2016. Available at: https://www.cdc.gov/nchs/data/nhis/earlyrelease/earlyrelease201605.pdf (accessed 1-182016).

[28] Eibner C, Saltzman (2015). How does the ACA individual mandate affect enrollment and premiums in the individual insurance market? RAND Research Brief. Available at: http://www.rand.org/pubs/research_briefs/RB981224.html (accessed 1-16-17).

only "small and inconsistent effects of the individual mandate in 2014 and 2015 with minimal policy impact."[29]

Regardless of the empirical evidence, the health insurance industry as well as health insurance experts have been clear for nearly three decades that some form of a coverage obligation is essential to provide a balanced risk pool and to provide necessary confidence that guaranteed issue can be maintained in a financially sustainable manner. A December 7 2016 letter to Speaker Paul Ryan and Leader Nancy Pelosi from the American Academy of Actuaries describes this dynamic well:

> "A sustainable health insurance market depends on enrolling enough healthy people over which the costs of the less healthy people can be spread. To ensure viability when there is a guarantee that consumers with pre-existing conditions can obtain health insurance coverage at standard rates requires mechanisms to spread the cost of that guarantee over a broad population. The ACA's individual mandate encourages even the young and healthy to obtain coverage."[30]

Among health insurance and health policy experts, widespread consensus exists that to maintain guaranteed issue without any pre-existing condition exclusions requires some enforceable mechanism to provide a robust and diverse risk profile among eligible consumers.

Second, to eliminate the mandate and leave in place guaranteed issue is a sure and proven formula for major disruption in the individual health insurance market nationally, a concern that is neither speculative nor hypothetical.

The experiences of states between the early 1990s and today demonstrates that the concern about the workability of guaranteed issue without some enforceable mechanism such as an individual mandate is a legitimate and essential issue. Eight states adopted guaranteed issue, most

---

[29] Frean M, Gruber J, Sommers BD (2016). Premium subsidies, the mandate and Medicaid expansion: coverage effects of the Affordable Care Act. NBER Working Paper 22213. Available at http://www.nber.org/papers/w22213.pdf (accessed 1-17-2017).

[30] Shari Westerfield. Letter from American Academy of Actuaries to Speaker Paul Ryan and Leader Nancy Pelosi. December 7 2016. Available at: http://actuary.org/files/publications/HPC_letter_ACA_CSR_120716.pdf (accessed 1-18-17).

during the 1990s. When the damage from guaranteed issue without some form of mandate became evident, some states abandoned the protections, while other states accepted the damage to their individual market risk pool and continued the practice.

As of 2012, only five states (Maine, Massachusetts, New Jersey, New York, and Vermont) required individual market health insurers to guarantee issue all products to all residents. These five states maintained their guaranteed issue requirements despite a collapse in participation by individual consumers in the face of growing unaffordable health insurance premiums. The impact was most dramatically evident in New York State where participation in the individual market dropped from 752,000 covered lives in the early 1990s when guaranteed issue was first adopted to about 34,000 covered lives in 2009.[31] Massachusetts saw a similar form of insurance "death spiral" when it adopted guaranteed issue in its individual health insurance market in 1996 without an accompanying mandate, only seeing the non-group market return to viability after implementation of the state's individual mandate in 2007.[32] Other states, notably New Hampshire, Kentucky, and Washington repealed or restricted their guaranteed issue rules once the market impact became clear. Four states (Michigan, Pennsylvania, Rhode Island, and Virginia, plus the District of Columbia) in 2012 still required their Blue Cross Blue Shield carrier to act as insurer of last resort, an increasingly unworkable formula as the cost of care for clients in the individual markets became increasingly unsustainable.[33]

Though guaranteed issue and the related banning of medical underwriting and pre-existing condition exclusions remain among the most popular features of the ACA, with public promises to retain it from President Trump, House Speaker Ryan, and Senate Majority Leader

---

[31] G. C. Sandler. "New York Individual Market Rules: The Nuts and Bolts of Rating in the Individual Market." National Health Policy Forum, Washington DC, February 19, 2009, slide 4.

[32] M. Hackmann et al. "Adverse Selection and an Individual Mandate: When Theory Meets Practice." American Economic Review. 2015 Mar; 105(3): 1030-66. Available at: https://www.ncbi.nlm.nih.gov/pmc/articles/PMC4408001/ (accessed 1-20-2017).

[33] Kaiser Family Foundation. "Health Insurance Market Reforms: Guaranteed Issue." Focus on Health Reform. June 2012. Available at: https://kaiserfamilyfoundation.files.wordpress.com/2013/01/8327.pdf (accessed 1-18-2017).

McConnell, the certain danger of maintaining guaranteed issue without an enforceable mandate of some form is neither speculative nor hypothetical. The Congressional Budget Office released a report as recently as January 17 concluding that "eliminating the mandate penalties and the subsidies while retaining the market reforms would destabilize the nongroup market and the effect would worsen over time."[34]

Third, between the late 1980s and 2009, the individual mandate was largely an idea championed by both conservative and moderate Republicans until former President Barack Obama endorsed it in June 2009.

The policy idea of a mandate on individuals to purchase health insurance as a mechanism to achieve near-universal coverage was introduced in the American health policy sphere in the late 1980s by Professor Mark Pauly of the University of Pennsylvania's Wharton School as an alternative to single-payer or employer mandate proposals to reach the same goal.[35] The idea was advanced and promoted by the Heritage Foundation, and especially by Dr. Stuart Butler, in the same period.[36] In the years 1993-1994 when the President Bill Clinton promoted national health reform legislation, Senators Robert Dole, John Chafee and Charles Grassley, along with 19 other Republican members of Congress as co-sponsors, advanced a proposal to establish a national mandate on most Americans to purchase health insurance as an alternative to the Clinton Administration's approach.[37] In the late 1990s, Louisiana Senator John Breaux became the first prominent Democrat to embrace the concept of the individual mandate.

---

[34] Congressional Budget Office. "How Repealing Portions of the Affordable Care Act Would Affect Health Insurance Coverage and Premiums." January 2017. Available at https://www.cbo.gov/sites/default/files/115th-congress2017-2018/reports/52371coverageandpremiums.pdf (accessed 1-18-2017).

[35] Pauly MV, Danzon P, Feldstein P and Hoff J (1991). A plan for 'responsible national health insurance.' Health Affairs 10(1): 5-25.

[36] Butler SM (1989). Assuring affordable health care for all Americans. Heritage Foundation. Accessed electronically 1/16/17 at http://www.heritage.org/research/lecture/assuring affordable-health-care-for-all-americans.

[37] M. Cooper. "Conservatives Sowed Idea of Health Care Mandate, Only to Spurn It Later." New York Time. February 14, 2012. Available at: http://www.nytimes.com/2012/02/15/health/policy/health-care-mandate-was-first-backed-byconservatives.html (accessed 1-18-2017).

In 2004, Massachusetts Governor Mitt Romney proposed legislation to establish a statewide individual mandate that drew support from overwhelming Democratic majorities in the State Senate and House of Representatives, from U.S. Senator Edward Kennedy, and from President George W. Bush whose Administration provided key financing for the program. The legislation was signed into law on April 12, 2006 in a ceremony in Boston's historic Faneuil Hall. Seated on the stage was a representative of the Heritage Foundation which consulted with Governor Romney on structuring the individual mandate and creating the Massachusetts Health Insurance Connector Authority, the first governmental example of a health insurance exchange, another concept championed by the Heritage Foundation.[38]

The Massachusetts law incorporated the "three-legged stool" concept that is the organizing idea behind Title 1 of the ACA: systemic insurance market reform including guaranteed issue, an individual mandate to purchase health insurance, and premium/cost sharing subsidies to make the buying of insurance affordable. When Governor Romney left his position in January 2007 to begin his first campaign for the Republican nomination for U.S. President, full implementation of the law was left to his successor, Gov. Deval Patrick. During Romney's 2008 campaign, he received the endorsement of Sen. James De Mint who noted in his letter of support that as Governor, Romney had "passed innovative health care reforms."[39]

During the 2008 campaign for the Democratic nomination for U.S. President, leading candidates Hillary Clinton and John Edwards both advanced health care reform proposals that included an individual mandate, while candidate Barack Obama did not. Indeed, President Obama did not officially endorse inclusion of an individual mandate in health reform legislation until June 2009, well after the Congressional process had started in earnest. It was in this period that many Congressional Republicans began to distance themselves from the individual mandate.

---

[38] P. Belluck and K. Zezima. "Massachusetts Legislation on Insurance Becomes Law." New York Times. Available at: http://www.nytimes.com/2006/04/13/us/13health.html (accessed 1-18-2017).

[39] H. Hewitt. "Senator Jim DeMint Endorses Romney." Available at: http://www.hughhewitt.com/senator-jim-demint-endorses-romney-he-is-strongly-pro-life/ (accessed 1-18-2016).

Exemplifying this change was Senator Charles Grassley who stated on Fox News in June 2009: "When it comes to states requiring it for automobile insurance, the principle then ought to lie the same way for health insurance because everybody has some health insurance costs, and if you aren't insured, there's no free lunch. Somebody else is paying for it."[40] Three months later, in September 2009, his views had shifted: "Individuals should maintain the freedom to choose whether to purchase health insurance coverage or not.[41]

Democrats embraced the individual mandate concept in the 2000s in good faith to find common ground on universal coverage with Republicans and conservatives on a key structural feature championed by the latter groups. But as the ground shifted for Democrats leading them to support the mandate was a practical way forward, the ground shifted for Republicans compelling them to abandon a policy they had themselves promoted for nearly two decades.

Fourth, other mechanisms could be used to replace the individual mandate, such as late enrollment penalties or the proposed "continuous coverage" requirement advanced in Speaker Paul Ryan's "Better Way" health proposal, though the latter requirement would be more punitive towards individual consumers than the ACA's individual mandate.

Several mechanisms have been proposed to replace the ACA's individual mandate in replacement legislation. One of these is a "late penalty" fee such as the ones included in Medicare Parts B and D.[42] The alternative most often advanced in recent months is the proposal that guaranteed issue only be applied to individuals who maintain "continuous coverage" of their health insurance policies within defined limits. This proposal received prominent backing in the House Republican

---

[40] Transcript: Sens. Dodd, Grassley on FNS. Fox News Sunday, June 14 2009. Available at: http://www.foxnews.com/story/2009/06/14/transcript-sens-dodd-grassley-on-fns.html (accessed 1-18-17).

[41] Live Pulse. "Grassley Backtracks on Individual Mandate." Politico. September 22 2009. Available at: http://www.politico.com/livepulse/0909/Grassley backtracks on individual mandate.html (accessed 1-18-2017).

[42] J. Holahan and L. Blumberg. "Instead of ACA Repeal and Replace, Fix it." Urban Institute. January 2017. Available at: http://www.urban.org/research/publication/instead-aca-repealand-replace-fix-it/view/fullreport (accessed 1-20-2017).

Leadership's "A Better Way" health proposals released this past June 2016:

> "Our plan also proposes a new patient protection for those Americans who maintain continuous coverage. ... If an individual experiences a qualifying life event, he or she would not be charged more than standard rates - even if he or she is dealing with a serious medical issue. ... However, making the decision to forego coverage during this one-time open enrollment period will result in the forfeiture of continuous coverage protections and lead to higher health insurance coverage costs for that individual for a period in the future."[43]

Individuals and families unable to avoid undefined coverage gaps permitted under the Better Way plan would be subject to medical underwriting and pre-existing condition exclusions for, as mentioned above, "a period in the future." Those individuals with any pre-existing conditions found to relevant by health insurance companies for underwriting purposes would be denied coverage. Under the Better Way plan, their recourse for denied insurance applicants would be to seek coverage from newly re-established state high risk pools. The experience with state high risk pools has been mixed at best. Pools first established in the 1970s were chronically underfunded, often with long waiting lists and high premiums, with coverage limits that were banned by the ACA, such as lifetime and annual benefit caps, waiting periods, and limited benefits.[44]

Beyond these concerns is the issue of just how many individuals would be newly subjected to what I refer to as the "medical underwriting circle of hell." The current estimate of uninsured Americans by the CDC is 29 million, while the CBO estimates that as many as 32 million Americans potentially losing their insurance under Republican repeal legislation vetoed by President Obama one year ago. While we can hope that any

---

[43] House of Representatives. "A Better Way: Our Vision for a Confidant America." June 2016. Available at: http://abetterway.speaker.gov/_assets/pdf/ABetterWay-HealthCarePolicyPaper.pdf (accessed 1-18-2017).

[44] K. Pollitz. "High Risk Pools for Uninsurable Individuals." Kaiser Family Foundation. August 1, 2016. Available at: http://kff.org/health-reform/issue-brief/high-risk-pools-for-uninsurableindividuals/ (accessed 1-18-2017).

ACA repeal will be accompanied by a robust replacement law that will fully cover all who may otherwise lose coverage, no such guarantee exists today. This new era of insurance industry medical underwriting will subject at least tens of millions of Americans to renewed medical underwriting. By comparison, in 2015 an estimated 7.5 million Americans paid the ACA individual mandate assessment on their tax return.[45]

Even though the health insurance industry has been vocal in advocating for changes to the ACA in line with its priorities, including for example repeal of the health insurance industry tax and adjustment to special enrollments periods, no leading industry voices have been urging the Congress or Administration to re-impose medical underwriting and pre-existing condition exclusions. My conversations with insurance industry executives reveal no desire to return to that sordid work. Americans take pride that the days of classifying our fellow citizens according to their medical histories are in the past, and they show no desire to return to them.

Fifth, no empirical evidence I can find suggests that the individual mandate is the cause of the stresses recently experienced during the 2017 enrollment cycle in some federal and state health insurance exchanges. Other causes more effectively explain these recent problems.

It is well known that many of the federal and state health insurance exchanges have experienced turbulent times leading up to 2017 enrollment year characterized by rising premiums and market disruption. Some suggest that problems with health exchanges in this period demonstrate a fatal marketplace meltdown, justifying calls to scrap the ACA's private insurance coverage structure and replace it with something new. It is a legitimate question - whether exchanges face fundamental dysfunction or temporary and fixable disruption. Regardless of one's conclusions on this question, no convincing evidence ties the disruption to the individual mandate. A related and legitimate question is whether the mandate's

---

[45] July 17 2016 letter from IRS Commissioner John Koskinen to Members of Congress. Available at: https://www.irs.gov/pub/irs-utl/CommissionerLetterlwithcharts.pdf (accessed 1-21-2017).

financial penalties are high enough - a question I will address in the next and final section.

Regarding the state of the ACA exchanges, a December 22 2016 "RatingsDirect" report from S&P Global concludes:

> "S&P Global Ratings expects U.S. health insurers to report improved underwriting performance in the individual market in 2016 versus 2015. Although most insurers will still report an underwriting loss for 2016, the losses will be smaller than in 2015. This means the changes made to network design and premium pricing are gaining traction, though more still needs to be done. For 2017, we expect continued improvement, with more insurers reporting close to break-even or better results for this segment."

S&P also believes that premium hikes for 2018 "will be well below the 2017 hike.[46] Despite the controversies over the future of the ACA and premium increases, signups in the 2016-17 open enrollment period were the most robust since the launch of the marketplaces in 2013-14.[47]

A noteworthy development involves the state of Alaska where, last spring, alarms sounded when premiums were projected to rise by more than 40% in the state's individual health insurance market. Rather than accept the increases, the Republican-controlled state legislature passed a law to establish a reinsurance mechanism for the individual market, a move that rapidly lowered premium increases to about 7%. The ACA included three recognized mechanisms to moderate premium growth: risk adjustment, reinsurance, and risk corridors. Under the ACA, the latter two expired after the first 3 years at the end of 2016, and the risk adjustment has been subject to controversial limitations imposed by the Congress.

---

[46] S&P Global Reports. "The ACA Individual Market: 2016 Will be Better Than 2015, But Achieving Target Profitability Will Take Longer." December 22, 2016. Available at: https://morningconsult.com/wp-content/uploads/2016/12/12-22-16-The-ACA-IndividualMarket-2016-Will-Be-Better-Than-2015-But-Achieving-Target-Profitability-Will-Take-Longer.pdf (accessed 1-18-2017).

[47] T. Jost. "HHS Sees Surge in Open Enrollment." Health Affairs Blog. December 22 2016. Available at: http://healthaffairs.org/blog/2016/12/22/aca-round-up-robust-marketplace enrollment-cbo-on-defining-health-insurance-and-more/ (accessed 1-20-2017).

These developments significantly exacerbated the 2016-17 turmoil in the ACA markets.

Beyond this, variation exists among the 51 state and federal exchanges, and a pattern emerges. Most states that have actively worked to make their exchanges succeed by meeting the needs of their citizens outperform exchanges where state political leaders have been antagonistic or apathetic to their success.

Sixth and finally, finally, the suggestion that the size of the individual mandate's tax penalty should be increased to enhance the uptake of individual health insurance is misguided. More effective would be increasing premium and cost sharing subsidies for income eligible consumers to more closely mirror affordability levels in the Massachusetts health insurance system.

Numerous commentators, inside and outside of the insurance industry, have suggested that the individual mandate is too weak to be effective and that the monetary penalty should be increased to provide a greater incentive to motivate individuals to purchase coverage.[48] The penalty for non-purchase of health insurance under the ACA applies to individuals and families deemed able to afford the cost. For 2017 and beyond, the penalty is $695 (adjusted for inflation in future years) or 2.5% of income, whichever is higher, for a full year without coverage. Under Massachusetts health reform, once fully implemented, the tax penalty for non-coverage reached a maximum of approximately $900 per year. Though different, the two sets of individual mandate penalties were fairly close in financial impact for non-coverage.

Once implemented, Massachusetts health reform triggered a major drop in the state's uninsurance rate from 7.7% in 2006 to 2.5% in 2015, and the rate had dropped to below 3% by 2008. Far more significant for Massachusetts than the size and scope of the individual mandate penalty was - and is the extent of premium and cost sharing subsidies available to eligible consumers. The Massachusetts affordability formula for eligible

---

[48] J. Goodman. "Six Problems with the ACA that Aren't Going Away." Health Affairs Blog. June 25, 2015. Available at: http://healthaffairs.org/blog/2015/06/25/six-problems-with-the-acathat-arent-going-away/ (accessed 1-19-2017).

consumers using the state's exchange is far more generous, as Table 1 below demonstrates:

Table 1. Individual Contributions to Subsidized Coverage under the 2006 MA Health Reform Law compared with the ACA, for Select Income Levels relative to the Federal Poverty Level

Income Relative to Poverty (%)	MA - Required contribution to subsidized single coverage as share of income (%)	ACA - Required contribution to subsidized coverage as share of income, 2015 (%)
100	0	2.01
150	0	4.02
200	2.1	6.30
250	3-4	8.10
300	4.2	9.56
350	No Cap	9.56
400	No Cap	9.56
Over 400	No Cap	No Cap

Source: Urban Institute.[49]

While not strictly comparable to Massachusetts, the current uninsurance rate for the U.S.is 8.6%.[50] Rather than increasing the size of the individual mandate tax penalty, more effective would be to address the reality that the affordability formulas for premium and cost sharing subsidies in the ACA is not generous enough for many families in the target income categories, most importantly for households with incomes over 250% of the Federal Poverty Line.

---

[49] L. Blumberg and J. Holahan. "After King v. Burwell: Next Steps for the Affordable Care Act." Urban Institute Research Report. August 2015. Available at: http://www.urban.org/sites/default/files/alfresco/publication-pdfs/2000328-After-King-v.Burwell-Next-Steps-for-the-Affordable-Care-Act.pdf (accessed 1-19-2017).

[50] R. Cohen et al. "Health Insurance Coverage: Early Release of Estimates from the National Health Interview Survey, January March 2016. National Center for Health Statistics. 9/2016. Available at: https://www.cdc.gov/nchs/data/nhis/earlyrelease/insur201609.pdf (accessed 1-19-2017).

Conclusion

Though the individual mandate is the most controversial and unpopular aspect of the ACA, it is a foundational element that enables the ACA to provide coverage to tens of millions of Americans who would otherwise be uninsured. It is also a key feature that permits the highly popular guaranteed issue rule to function effectively. Removing the individual mandate by itself would have negative consequences for the health security of many tens of millions of Americans and would move our nation backwards in terms of addressing the key challenges we face in continuously improving our nation's health and health care.

Chairman BUCHANAN. I want to thank all of you. It is excellent testimony. We now proceed to questions and answer session. For the purposes of today's hearing, I will hold my question until the end.

I will now recognize the gentleman from Pennsylvania, Mr. Meehan.

Mr. MEEHAN. Thank you, Mr. Chairman and the Ranking Member. And I am going to look forward to working with both of you and the full Committee on this important agenda before us. And there couldn't be a more appropriate place to start than with this particular issue.

One of the concerns that I hear back in my district frequently is the frustration of everyday Americans with Federal Government mandates telling people this is the way you are going to live your lives. It would be bad enough if that was all that there was to it. But the fact of the matter is we are talking about something which, notwithstanding the opening statement of my good friend the Ranking Member, the ACA does not work. And I was pleased to see Mr. Miller talk about the concept of exposed nerves from the Federal mandates that are happening. And we hear words about mandate, coercion. Those are the kinds of things that I think are affecting people.

And then you look at the facts. We have had this program. Premiums have been rising by double digits for the very people that Mr. McDonough talked about in the hardest places to be able to pay. One-third of the counties now have only a single insurer. The exchanges are consisting largely now of older and less healthy people.

And I look at my own district in Pennsylvania. And we have taken the time to ask people to weigh in. Premiums for ObamaCare plans of Pennsylvania are up 33 percent in 2017. Each year there is fewer to choose from. In 2016, there were 13 plans. Next year, there will be eight. Now listen to the individuals in their own words. Mike from Boyertown shared with me his concern, the cost of our health care insurance. "We have coverage from healthcare.gov and our rates are increasing from $1,600 to $2,600 a month." These are working class people. "Only six plans are available, and the lowest cost one is still over $2,000 per month just for my wife and I." Fred from Lansdale wrote, "I received my annual health insurance rate increase for 2017 yesterday. My rates went up from $2,500 to over $3,750 per month. Per month. Last year's increase was devastating. This year's increase is even more overwhelming. I am self-employed. I only had a few short years ago. This news is devastating to my family."

People are voting with their feet in this. The CBO just came out and released its most recent, just this week. Expects a sharply lower number of participants in the Affordable Care Act for exchanges in 2017. CBO said the number of participants in the exchange was expected to be 10 million in 2017. So clearly, we have been sold a bill of goods. It isn't working.

Mr. Miller, what conclusions can you draw from this kind of revised estimate?

Mr. MILLER. Well, it is not working according to plan is the short answer. To connect this up with the subject of today's hearing, one of this—this reflects, in effect, an overinvestment in a set of policies that did not come together and work as promised. And part of what you are seeing in the higher premiums and the restricted availability of plans, the losses in plans, is everybody was supposedly saying it is all going to work like clockwork. Everybody is going to go into the exchanges. That is what CBO projected. They weren't talking to the people on the ground. And so we have got a different experience in practice than the one that was proposed to us in theory.

Now, we can keep trying to implement that theory saying sooner later it will work out. That seems to be what CBO is mostly projecting. On the other hand, we can try to say we need to take this into the shop and change the mix around. And we need to get back to having health care coverage that actually matches what people are willing to pay for and can pay for.

Mr. MEEHAN. I am so glad you said that about taking it into the shop. Because here is the big misnomer in this whole discussion. This idea that somehow there is this Republican effort to just drop the thing and leave everybody on the street, instead of the real genuine effort which is to take something that isn't working and try to get it to work better.

We only get 40 percent of the people who are eligible for these exchanges into it. And yet we need about 72 percent to make them work. So how do we incent that other 30 percent to get in? Is it by mandates or is it by working on the kinds of things which are being put in place to lower the cost, to make better availability, to make their—allow the programs to be the kinds of things in which they have a choice to find the insurance that fits them? Isn't that the better way to get that remaining 30 percent so we can get the kind of exchanges that can actually work?

Mr. MILLER. We have tried the weak punitive approach or we know what is best. We might want to try some positive incentives to find out what in fact—where the market is.

Mr. MEEHAN. Mr. Chairman, thank you. I yield back.

Chairman BUCHANAN. I now want to recognize the distinguished Ranking Member, Mr. Lewis, for any question he might have.

Mr. LEWIS. Thank you very much, Mr. Chairman.

Dr. McDonough, one of the things I am most proud of in today's law is that because of the ACA, Americans with preexisting conditions are able to get insurance. Can you discuss why the individual mandate is so necessary?

Mr. MCDONOUGH. So thank you for the question, Representative. The concept of guaranteed issue, which means that insurers must issue coverage to applicants regardless of their prior medical history, regardless of their current medical status, is one of the most popular features of the Affordable Care Act. It is a policy that was implemented in various States starting in the 1990s. About eight States in particular. Five States implemented it. All eight States implemented it without an individual mandate. And all States, when they did it, saw significant substantial disruption in their individual health insurance market because people were going in and purchasing coverage when they felt they need it and then dropping out of the market when they got whatever services they needed.

And so it was a damaging risk pool that created what some refer to as an insurance death spiral where premiums go up, and as premiums go up, more people drop out. We saw that in Massachusetts, New York, New Jersey, Vermont, and other States. Kentucky, New Hampshire. Some States did guaranteed issue without a mandate. And when they saw the impact, they withdrew and they stopped guaranteed issue. Other States, like Massachusetts and New York, did it and had damaging impacts in the market and kept the policy in place.

But guaranteed issue is one of the most popular features of the law. Americans don't like the idea that to get coverage you can only get it if you don't have any adverse medical history that would disqualify you from coverage. And they don't like the individual mandate. And they usually don't understand that there is a link between the two of them. And that guaranteed issue can't function effectively in an environment without some kind of coverage responsibility, some kind of shared responsibility on the part of individuals. So that is where it comes from, and so—the linking together.

And so Massachusetts, in 2006, in its Health Insurance Reform Law, for the first time put together and actually implemented an individual mandate and guaranteed issue together. We saw a dramatic drop in our rate of uninsurance. We saw a stabilization, a stabilization of premiums in the individual market. And it was a strikingly successful experiment in terms of the intended influence on the individual health insurance marketplace. So we saw it at work.

And it was then the design feature that people thought made sense in terms of coming up with the national reform that is the Affordable Care Act. So that's where it came from and that is why it is in there. It is an essential piece. So Americans love guaranteed issue and don't want to lose that. But guaranteed issue without some kind of coverage requirement creates a serious market disruption which people would not want to see.

Mr. LEWIS. Thank you very much, Doctor. Would you talk about the best ways to get people enrolled in insurance and engaged in their health care? Is it better to increase financial assistance or to follow the Republican suggestion such as the Better Way health proposal?

Mr. MCDONOUGH. So the concern that I have with the Better Way health proposal and with some of the other plans that are forward is that, you know, the United States in January 1, 2014, banished medical underwriting from our health insurance market for the first time in our history. And overwhelmingly Americans like that reform. Don't want to go back. And that seems to be fairly bipartisan.

The concern that I see in terms of the suggestion to have guaranteed issue but only for people who can maintain continuous coverage is that there will literally be, in a very short period of time, tens of millions of Americans who will then fall back into the circle of people who will be newly subject to medical underwriting and have their insurance-ability, their ability to buy insurance, rated based upon their medical history. I think that would be a terribly unfortunate step backward that Americans would not appreciate and have rejected that approach.

Mr. LEWIS. And thank you very much, Doctor.

I yield back.

Chairman BUCHANAN. I now recognize Mr. Smith from Missouri.

Mr. SMITH. Thank you, Mr. Chairman.

Back in December, I held health care roundtables throughout our congressional district in southeast and south central Missouri to just hear from farmers, small business owners, families of the experiences that they have had under ObamaCare. And the message was very consistent. Forcing citizens to buy a product they simply didn't want or suffer a tax penalty is un-American, especially when in many cases that product is too expensive and not adequate.

As the gentleman from Pennsylvania mentioned briefly of the exchanges in his State going from 13 to 8 I think were the numbers, out of the 30 counties in the Eighth Congressional District of Missouri, individuals who are forced under the individual mandate, you know what their options are? Out of 30 counties, 26 of those 30 counties has one choice. Looks like adequate options. Absolutely not. Take the case of Doug from southeast Missouri. He is a 61- year-old divorced cabinetmaker who helps his 20-year-old daughter and ex-wife pay for their health insurance. Doug started a small business just over 3 years ago. He wrote me. This is what he wrote: "My business is beginning to be profitable. However, with startup costs and normal business costs, cash flow, et cetera, there is nothing left of the budget for my personal health insurance. I have been without coverage for 2-1/2 years. I make too much to qualify for subsidies, not that I would take advantage anyway, and do not make enough to pay the premiums after paying for everyone else. The ACA penalty adds injury to insult. Insult because the whole mandated mess is unconstitutional. And injury because I usually have to take out yet another business loan to pay my income taxes after the ACA penalty."

I checked prices for insurance for a 61-year-old man in his county of Missouri, and it is somewhere in the neighborhood of $900 a month. That is more than the typical rent payment in southeast Missouri and would likely represent one of the largest expenses he would be paying. So who is the policy really helping, I ask? It is definitely not the lower and middle class in southeast Missouri. The mandate targets individuals, but it also hurts the health care facilities and hospitals who help serve them.

During one of our roundtables, the Chief Executive Officer of one of the federally qualified health centers testified that in their area, 37.3 percent of the population they serve are uninsured. But yet everyone is required to have health insurance under the individual mandate.

The mandate was designed to address uncompensated care, but it didn't. Here is the bottom line. ObamaCare's individual mandate has failed. Special enrollment periods and exemptions by the Obama Administration created an environment that goes completely against the idea of a mandate that created an unfair burden on facilities in my district that offer care to low-income individuals.

My question is to Mr. Miller. Your testimony highlighted weak enforcement and weak compliance as challenges with the individual mandate. Can you explain in more detail how the individual mandate harms the low- and middle-income people it was supposedly designed to help?

Mr. MILLER. Well, I am trying to go backwards from where you are talking about. Part of it is because it didn't deliver what it said it was going to do. In terms of the coverage effects you saw, where those people went was primarily into Medicaid to the extent they were lower income. That is what they ended up choosing rather than the exchange-based coverage. And that is where they have ended up. However, insurers along the way have incurred some substantial losses within these exchange markets because their original business plans assumed a different set of enrollment and a different level of compliance with a mandate which was never enforced in that manner. So that the mismatch has created, in effect, a compression of plans and the rising premiums. There are other distinctions along the way.

Some of the statements that have been made about the scope of uncompensated care costs, if you look at the vast historical record, vastly exaggerated. Now, this law has a lot of moving parts. We took away some of the funding for that uncompensated care as— on the assumption it was going to be made up for by the increased enrollment. That didn't match up. We have had behavioral changes which indicate that people who are nominally insured are still going to emergency rooms anyway.

So it is hard to isolate the mandate alone along this broader mosaic of basically a floundering law which has many different theories behind it that don't work out in practice.

Mr. SMITH. Thank you, Mr. Chairman.

Chairman BUCHANAN. I now recognize the gentleman from New York, Mr. Crowley.

Mr. CROWLEY. Thank you, Mr. Chairman. Thanks very much. I appreciate this hearing today.

If I can, I just want to—my good friend, I mean this with all sincerity, from Pennsylvania. I think the world of Pat Meehan and he knows it. He made the reference at the end of his comments where this notion or idea come from that Republicans want to repeal without replacing. And I would just note for the record that we have had 65 attempts to repeal the

Affordable Care Act, or ObamaCare, over the last 6 or so years without ever once offering a replacement. Maybe that is where we might get the idea that you simply want—you all simply want to repeal the bill without replacing it. That is just an observation.

Mr. McDonough, my home State of New York provides a valuable example of how the requirement to buy insurance is a critically important aspect of the ACA to provide stability in the individual insurance market. Before the ACA, New York's individual market did not include an individual mandate. So the market did not have enough healthy individuals. As a result, monthly individual premiums reached over $1,500 and less than 20,000 people had enrolled.

Now as a result of the Affordable Care Act, premiums for individuals are 50 percent lower than they would have been without the ACA. The number of New Yorkers in the individual market has grown by 270 percent. And plan participation in more—is more robust. Sixteen insurers offer coverage in the individual market and 21 serve the small group market.

Mr. McDonough, would you say that New York's experience with the mandate illustrates just why it is so critical and the dangers that could happen if it is repealed or undermined?

Mr. MCDONOUGH. So thank you, Representative, for that question. I think it is important to recognize that the issues with the Federal and State health insurance exchanges from New York, from Pennsylvania, from Missouri, from all of the different States vary. So there are some States that are going through very significant disruption and very critically high rises in premiums. There are other States like, for example, New York and California, that are doing very well actually in terms of a moderate rate of growth.

There is the striking example that we have of the State of Alaska. Alaska last spring had projections that the premiums in their individual market were going to go up by over 40 percent. In the summer, the Alaska legislature with their governor agreed to create a reinsurance pool within the State individual health insurance market just in Alaska. When they did that, that single act, they brought their projected premium increases from 40 percent down to 7 percent.

So part of the difference, and it is not exclusively this, but it is very much a factor, part of the difference is that States that have aggressively grabbed and worked to take a leadership role in helping this new health insurance market to work and succeed have seen strikingly better results in terms of premium growth and in terms of plan participation than States that have, for their own legitimate reasons, been very hostile to the implementation and have had not only nothing that they wanted to do to help it, but actually worked consciously and proactively to try to undermine the implementation of the law.

So there is a real difference there. And I think it is worth understanding that you can make differences happen here. States need to be part of the solution. And the States that have done that have made a real difference. Sorry for too much time in that answer.

Mr. CROWLEY. That is all right.

Mr. Chairman, I have a letter from the Department of Financial Services in New York State which oversees the insurance industry in the State. I would just ask that we include that for the record to the Committee.

Chairman BUCHANAN. Yeah, that is fine.

Mr. CROWLEY. I just wanted to say, listen, this is incredibly complicated, all the parts that go into making the Affordable Care Act work itself. We talked about, you know, the mandates. We haven't talked about other aspects that have—in the whole, that make it actually work or in theory work. So, listen, I understand the frustration. We have been frustrated for the last 6 years. We haven't found any partners to actually improve the Act as opposed to just repealing it.

I think my colleagues on the other side of the aisle realize now, as does the new President, how difficult it is to take away the sweets. It is the vegetables, I think, my colleagues have had a difficult time swallowing in order to get to the sweets first. But I think they are learning that. And I yield back.

Chairman BUCHANAN. I now recognize the gentleman from Arizona, Mr. Schweikert.

Mr. SCHWEIKERT. Thank you, Mr. Chairman. And those of us with a sweet tooth, we will work on that. And, Mr. Chairman and fellow Members and obviously the panel, being from Arizona, when you use the term "disruption," we're one of the epicenters of it. You know, if it wasn't for almost a charitable gift by I think our Blue Cross Blue Shield going into a couple counties, I would have had counties—remember, my State has only 15 counties. So our counties are huge. They would have had no offering.

So could I beg of you, and this is going to be a little different, but this is something staff and I have been trying to hunt for years. Could we do a little math together? I need some help on something. What I am hunting for is—and we have even had researchers from Kaiser and other people try to help us. And the Administration has been willfully difficult, and maybe it is because the way the data sets are collected. Maybe it is obfuscation. Maybe it is perfectly innocent.

If I go back at the end of fiscal year 2016, we functionally have had what? Three years out there where there was product offered. How many of our brothers and sisters gained coverage that either did not have coverage before or who were not Medicaid eligible? And when I say did not have coverage before, truly had gone long term. Not where they had 3 days between jobs and we called them uncovered. But how many—I mean, what is the real number? How many folks now have coverage by the end of fiscal year 2016 that did not have any either access to coverage or weren't Medicaid eligible? And can anyone give me an honest number? This is an open—I mean, this is a fly ball for whoever can pitch it back.

Mr. MILLER. I don't usually like to do this in a hearing. I may have to quote Jon Gruber. And I only do that every couple of years. Because even a stopped clock may be right a couple of times a day.

Based on those recent calculations, approximately 60 percent of the coverage gains came from Medicaid. There is a little bit of a dispute as to how much of that is expansion Medicaid and how much of that is old Medicaid.

Mr. SCHWEIKERT. Look, we have 2 minutes and 30 seconds to play here. So, okay, let's say it is 60 percent of the population gained it through

Medicaid. Then of the remaining 40, I have seen some numbers out there that say a substantial portion of that had either access to or had coverage at some time before. And my——

Mr. MILLER. Some of that is old Medicaid. There is a provision where if you go into the hospital, you can get signed up for Medicaid. That is under old Medicaid as well as new Medicaid. There were States who were already expanding before 2014. It makes that old Medicaid.

Mr. SCHWEIKERT. So is it——

Mr. MILLER. Some of it came from the individual exchanges, though. That is a fact.

Mr. SCHWEIKERT. Okay. So who——

Mr. MILLER. But probably about only about half of the exchange coverage more or less are actually net uninsured getting coverage.

Some of them were people who got pushed out of the other part of the individual market.

Mr. SCHWEIKERT. And, look, I understand this is a little difficult and there is a lot of moving parts here. As someone just said, it is complicated. So are we now down to 7 million?

Mr. MILLER. We could be down to 6 or 7 million. And, again, these are fuzzy numbers because we pretend that our data is excellent and you can raise four or five different surveys and get different numbers and make different assumptions.

Mr. SCHWEIKERT. In the next minute and 30 seconds, let's pretend we are accountants. Okay. So over the beginning of this law till the end of 2016, how much has been spent? And when I say "spent," I mean by the Federal Government, the State government, individual premiums, losses from insurance companies, others. What is my total dollar amount? Because I have seen numbers at, you know, $500 billion. I mean, I have seen some really interesting numbers that if you do a true all-in math, and I am—you see where I am going. For 3 years of coverage, my all-in cost to help 7 million, I could almost do that in the top of my head. Someone is going to correct me later. $68,000 per life? I mean, I am buying their health coverage, and I could have probably bought them a really nice car.

So something's wrong. And just if we take a step backwards, whether it be the individual mandate or just the basic math of if we all agreed we want to help our brothers and sisters out there, our total dollars per total life coverage, something is horribly wrong in what we are doing. Am I being unfair?

Mr. MCDONOUGH. I would just respond, Mr. Schweikert, by saying that I think that 6 million is a significant understatement. And I don't want to put out a number that I can't defend.

Mr. SCHWEIKERT. Okay. I would be elated if you could do me one of the grandest favors of all. Because we really—and my staff is back there laughing at me. I have spent a couple years of my life looking for this number, and talking to really smart people like yourself. Help me find real math. Because I come from a world of the math is the math is the math. But right now I am looking at numbers where I could have bought their coverage and bought them a nice car. Something's horribly wrong in what we're doing.

Thank you. And I yield back, Mr. Chairman.

Mr. MCDONOUGH. Happy to do that, sir.

Chairman BUCHANAN. I now recognize the gentlewoman from Indiana, Mrs. Walorski.

Mrs. WALORSKI. Thank you, Mr. Chairman.

President Obama promised over and over again, if you like your doctor, you can keep your doctor. If you like your health plan, you can keep your health plan. And despite these repeated pledges, we know now that these statements were completely untrue. In fact, in the fall of 2013, millions of Americans started receiving plan cancellation notices. PolitiFact ranked President Obama's statement as its lie of the year in 2013. But it wasn't just the immediate loss of plans. People are still losing them. For example, in Indiana last year, four insurers left the exchange, leaving Hoosiers with fewer options. That is 50 percent loss of our own plans. Recently, I heard from a constituent of mine from Starke County in Indiana.

He has had two open heart surgeries at Mayo Clinic that requires him to be on blood thinning and other medications, as well as periodic checkups. He had a private health insurance plan that he liked. Covered his medical needs. But in 2015, it was knocked out by ObamaCare. He was forced to buy a health care policy on the marketplace, but unfortunately discovered at an annual checkup at Mayo Clinic that his doctors were not in the network. And because of that and because they were out of State, they were out. He was forced to pay thousands of dollars out of pocket for the visit, in addition to thousands more out of pocket for the prescriptions. When he appealed to the Indiana Department of Insurance, he was told there was no marketplace insurance plan that would cover his doctors at Mayo Clinic as a Hoosier living in the State of Indiana.

He recently learned that his marketplace plan through UnitedHealthcare won't offer individual market plans for his area in 2017. He was forced back into the marketplace again to find a new health care plan that still will not cover his out-of-state doctors. It reinforces to me that for many Americans, this law is not working as promised.

And Mr. Miller and Mr. Graham, I wanted to direct this to you. Isn't it true that the individual mandate was supposed to increase competition on the exchanges by ensuring that people sign up, thereby encouraging insurance carriers to offer more choices and broaden those networks?

Mr. GRAHAM. That was the stated objective. And as you have described it, it has not been the case. So I agree, I guess, would be my answer.

Mrs. WALORSKI. Mr. Miller.

Mr. MILLER. As I like to say, it seemed like a good idea at the time. Although, unlike Mr. McDonough's testimony, it has been a bad idea for many of us for a long period of time on the conservative Republican side of the aisle, just to rewrite history a little bit, going back to the 1990s.

What was proposed wasn't executed. And it wasn't going to work that way because of the grand design, in theory, did not reflect the reality on the ground. Some people gained under this arrangement. There is no question about that. If you were a low-income person suddenly getting substantial subsidies for coverage, you might not be crazy about that coverage, but you will say you came out ahead. There are other people in that market, though, who had something that they were comfortable with or at least were ready to settle for. They were told that is not good enough. These are the folks who got moved out of other parts of the individual market and ended up with less effective choices and ones they didn't want. And that is what you are mostly hearing from among your constituents.

Mr. GRAHAM. And that is not going to turn around on its own. I think President Obama's Council of Economic Advisers just before they left asserted that the insurers have now got it figured out, everything is under control. The first 3 years you had the training wheels on board and—but now we are good to go. That doesn't make any sense. You know, the last year, from 2016 to 2017, you had by far the worst premium increase, 25 percent nationwide average. It is not getting better, it is getting worse. It is like the insurers are having more and more trouble every year they stay in the exchange.

Mrs. WALORSKI. Well, I guess my follow-up is, when insurance networks have become so narrow that individuals like my constituent, and there is many of those in Indiana, I just talked about one. When they lose access to their doctors, what does that say about the individual mandate's effectiveness to begin with?

Mr. GRAHAM. I think it says you are on the route to Medicaid for everybody where there is very poor access to care in many cases. So folks like—I know some of the Members have given testimony from their constituents. The whole structure is so terrible. You know, you earn an income that is—you are not Medicaid eligible so you can't even get the poor access to care that Medicaid offers. You might get some tax credit in the ObamaCare. Maybe you make too much money for that. Hard work to figure all that out, you know. And then the IRS comes after you next year and says you owe money back. So the complexity is far too complex. And I think when you go from one insurer to no insurer, as in Arizona, you were very lucky. I mean, what is a market where there is no insurance offered? It is not a market.

Mrs. WALORSKI. Right. I appreciate it.

Mr. Chairman, I yield back.

Chairman BUCHANAN. I now recognize the gentleman from Illinois, Mr. Davis.

Mr. DAVIS. Thank you very much, Mr. Chairman. And I want to thank all of our witnesses who are being very helpful as we deal with one of the most complex issues and problems that I think we face today as it relates to health care.

I represent the State of Illinois in the seventh district, which contains more hospital beds than any other congressional district in the country. The Affordable Care Act, which also has been beneficial to the four major medical center operations, medical schools that we are all so fortunate to have, the Affordable Care Act has greatly improved access to care for tens of millions of Americans. Enrollees now have access to medical homes, in general no longer have to rely solely on hospital emergency rooms, and have the comfortability of knowing that when they need care, it is available there for them.

Today, more than 1 million Illinoisans have health insurance coverage as a result of ACA, either due to the law's Medicaid expansion or its health insurance marketplace, and the majority of whom were uninsured prior to September 2013 when the ACA's coverage expansions were first implemented. Because of ACA the Nation's insurance uninsured population has dropped dramatically to less than 11 percent currently from nearly 17 percent in 2013.

If Congress repeals health insurance coverage, Illinois would sustain a potential loss of $11.6 billion, $13.1 billion in annual economic activity, and about 95,000 jobs lost. Ultimately, any attempt to repeal the ACA should be accompanied with an appropriate and responsible replacement plan that, at a minimum, ensures access to coverage for the more than 20 million U.S. residents who now have coverage as a result of the law.

If Congress does not make repeal of coverage contingent on adoption of an ACA replacement plan, then lawmakers should also correspondingly repeal the significant hospital payment cuts that help pay for ACA's coverage expansions. This is important for Illinois's hospitals and health systems which, to date, have had to absorb the more than $1 billion in Medicare reimbursement cuts to pay for the cost of the law's coverage expansion. For example, Northwestern Medical has seven hospitals alone, including Northwestern Memorial Hospital. They have absorbed more than $273 million in Medicare cuts since 2011.

Mr. McDonough, can you see institutions sustaining those kind of cuts and expenditures and continue to provide the level of care and service that they currently provide?

Mr. MCDONOUGH. Thank you, Mr. Davis. And no, I don't see that. I think there is a real difference across the country right now in terms of the financial health of hospitals, frankly between States that have expanded Medicaid under the ACA and States that have not. The States that have expanded along with the robust expansions through the marketplace have seen much greater financial health. And in States that have not expanded, there has been a far higher rate of hospital closure and of serious financial dilemma facing hospitals and other medical providers in those States. So it is a real difference and an indicator of what may come were there to be total repeal. Sorry.

Mr. DAVIS. Thank you.

Thank you, Mr. Chairman.

Chairman BUCHANAN. I now recognize the gentleman from Florida, Mr. Curbelo.

Mr. CURBELO. Mr. Chairman, thank you very much for holding this hearing. It will be my honor to serve under you in this Congress and with my colleagues here, especially Ranking Member Mr. Lewis, who I was proud to welcome to my community recently to celebrate Dr. Martin Luther King Day. And I also want to thank the witnesses for their testimony today.

Dr. McDonough, we share someone in common, Dr. Julio Frenk was the dean at your school. He has since moved up in the world, transferring to the University of Miami where he serves as president, which happens to be my alma mater.

Mr. Chairman, although enrollment in the ACA is relatively high in Florida, particularly in the Miami-Dade metropolitan area, choices continue to decrease and premiums continue to rise. This year, the counties in my district have lost insurance carriers. Monroe County lost one carrier and Miami-Dade lost two carriers participating on the exchange. I have heard people in my district about how the current system has reduced their choices and increased their out-of-pocket costs.

Emily, my constituent, explained that she is paying over $700 per month for a plan with a deductible that is over $6,000. But still she has been unable to find a doctor in her area who will accept her insurance. Even though she has insurance, her options are severely limited and premiums continue to increase.

Mr. Miller, I have a question for you. These examples that you have heard here today, and I think it is important that we raise them because statistics are fundamental to understanding what is happening in the world, but these real life human examples matter also. Do you believe that these examples are isolated, unique to our districts or are these the types of things that are happening all over the country?

Mr. MILLER. Well, there is a battle of warring anecdotes and everybody has to have their respective horror story, and you can get them on both sides. In the aggregate, though, we know that this is not working out in reaching its residual level. I comment somewhat in light of some of the discussions here that I am surprised that this embrace by folks who are more favorable to the Affordable Care Act of what you might think of as trickle-down economics. Let's first take care of the hospitals, let's first take care of the insurers, and maybe some people on the ground might eventually get some benefit from this.

This was a very interesting academic study of the Medicare expansion population, one showing that it had grown quite larger in terms of the cost per capita for the new adult, newly eligible able-bodied adults, but it hasn't necessarily delivered any more services. There is another study that indicated the Medicaid beneficiaries actually valued the coverage they received at about 20 to 40 cents on the dollar. So we are pumping more money into the system, but it isn't necessarily getting down to the ground level where it is actually improving people's care. And that is because the system is designed not for the beneficiaries at the end of it to be calling the shots, but somewhere along the line we determined what is good for them and what they should receive. And it works for other people in the system;

doesn't necessarily deliver that value at the bottom line for the consumers we supposedly care about.

Mr. CURBELO. So, Mr. Miller, are you suggesting that perhaps major health care special interests such as hospital chains, insurance companies and pharmaceuticals were too influential in the drafting of the last health care reform legislation?

Mr. MILLER. The previous Administration had to cut a deal and in some cases they had to give as well as take. And part of that deal was to make sure that they had placated those interests first in order to get the legislation passed.

Mr. CURBELO. Mr. Graham, with regards to the individual mandate, some suggest, well, this is, as we have kind of concluded here, not working very well, perhaps the solution is to raise the penalty and coerce more people into signing up for health insurance. I don't think that would be a very popular measure, and I assume most Members of this Committee and in this House would probably not be predisposed to supporting that kind of measure. What are some alternatives?

Mr. GRAHAM. I think Mr. Miller proposed some good alternatives. I think Professor McDonough's criticisms of those alternatives is also valid. There is a certain population, if you are just going to say you have got to maintain continuous coverage, you have got to—or pay a fine or whatever, there is some level of population that will not pay that. This is just a reality.

You know, when you lose your job, your mortgage payment or your rent comes first and you are going to drop your health insurance premiums. So there will always be some population that has to—you know, I hate to say it—be taken care of, but the social safety net. And I know on your side of the aisle you have talked about high risk pools, things like that.

I would just like to point out that, you know, Massachusetts had a reform that had some good things, some bad some things, the gentleman from New York who has left, every State had all these tools at their disposal. So what I would like to say is if we don't know the perfect answer, the magic bullet, let's let 50 States try and figure it out and learn from them.

Mr. CURBELO. Thank you. I yield back.

Chairman BUCHANAN. I now recognize the gentleman from North Carolina, Mr. Holding.

Mr. HOLDING. Thank you, Mr. Chairman.

I am going to pick up where my colleague, Mr. Meehan, left off. He listed some good testimony regarding the mandate not panning out, producing the numbers. We have got a slide, if we could put up there, of ACA exchange enrollment expectations versus reality. There. And you have done a good job of talking about some of the problems with the mandate. But it is clear that the economic modeling that the Obama Administration was using, they overestimated the strength of the mandate.

So perhaps, Mr. Miller, you could pick up here. Why would the models overestimate the mandate strengths so pretty dramatically there?

Mr. MILLER. I would say the first reason is they relied upon evidence from Massachusetts and Massachusetts' experts, which was unique to Massachusetts as opposed to the rest of the country. And that was built into a lot of the over assumptions of the high yield from the mandate. They also assumed they would have larger effects further up the scale. And the reality is if you subsidize people heavily, as turned out to be the case for basically those below 200 percent of Federal poverty level, you will get a lot of people, even though they are not crazy about the coverage, they will take it because it doesn't cost them much of anything when you add in the cost-sharing subsidies. You've got a lot of complaints about high deductibles. That has differential effects because of the way in which those cost-sharing subsidies in the exchanges tend to mute those out.

So when you were trying to get more people to come into this market who are either younger or had a little bit more money or were healthier, it turned out it was a bad deal for them. There's plenty of work done by some economists at the University of Pennsylvania, Wharton School, which talked about why you just didn't pay for people to take this coverage compared to either paying a penalty or dodging it in one form or another.

So all of this idea that new revenue was going to come in to pay for what we wanted didn't work out that way. And some of that is reflected in the reduced enrollment that was assumed but never materialized because you run out of subsidies to pay for people. And when it turns out that people have to pay for something they don't want, they don't buy it.

Mr. HOLDING. Right. Well, you know, speaking of subsidies, I find it kind of remarkable that according to some estimates that we have seen, that only about 40 percent of the subsidy eligible population signed up on the exchange. Now, this is concerning. I mean, do you find it concerning and why do you think it is?

Mr. MILLER. Well, that reflects the fact that as you move further up the ladder beyond what I just cited, which is about 60 to 65 percent, those subsidies aren't particularly generous. They are there, but they begin to phase out. This is a highly skewed, very progressive, if you want to use that term, approach to subsidizing very low-income individuals, even more so in the Medicaid-eligible population.

So mission accomplished in terms of getting that target population, but it didn't fit into the larger economic model which assumed that somewhere there was something else to pay for this. They tried a lot of other gimmicks in order to do this, but it didn't actually materialize in the way in which it was originally designed. And part of that is because it was a built-in ceiling on how much the individual mandate could ever produce, despite all the theories to the contrary, and also how much money that was actually there to subsidize people. And we found out that we are going to have come up with some other solutions.

Mr. HOLDING. Well, you know, you have got the benefit now of some history; you know, you have got a graph, we have got some real numbers in. And, you know, you mentioned at the top of the hearing in your prepared remarks, you know, the CBO is doubling down on these flawed estimates. I mean, what would the rationale be behind that?

Mr. MILLER. Well, people when they do models have assumptions and they tend to not want to let go of them. There are some things external to what originally started out that are moved around. Certainly, the Supreme Court decision changed some of the projections in terms of Medicaid enrollment. But the ingrained view that somehow the individual mandate was going to draw in all these people and they were going to comply and was going to be enforced didn't work out that way.

Potentially by some, you know, standard you could have about— you know, at one time they had a 30-million target population, and it turned out that only 3 million of those people were actually—you know, were paying into the individual mandate as opposed to staying uninsured. It is the difference between theory and practice. We have learned a lot about theories. We need to go back to reexamining what will work in practice.

Mr. HOLDING. Thank you very much.

Mr. Chairman, I yield back.

Chairman BUCHANAN. We have been joined at this hearing by our fellow Ways and Means Committee Member, Mr. Kelly. As is our custom, he will be permitted to ask witnesses questions. Now that the Members of the Subcommittee have concluded their questioning, Mr. Kelly from Pennsylvania, you are now recognized for 5 minutes.

Mr. KELLY. Thank you, Chairman. And again, thank you for allowing me to participate today.

All three of you are here for a reason. We talked today the purpose of the hearing is to examine if the individual mandate penalty is actually stabilizing health markets. Okay? And we talked about a lot of different things. I have got so many constituents back home that now have a policy, but don't have any health care.

So between premiums being where they are, deductibles being where they are, copays being where they are, I know there is reference made to Medicaid. The question is who all accepts Medicaid as payment? How many actual providers of health care say, no thanks, it doesn't begin to cover my cost of delivery?

So here is what it comes down to. If we are talking about this and if a big part of the individual mandate was going to cover the cost of all these things, the question is did it work? Is there anybody of the three of you that could say this was—it was well intended? I am going to say it wasn't well intended.

And, Mr. Miller, I love the fact it is three versus practice. Again, it is assuming things without looking at reality. People usually don't buy things they don't want and they certainly don't overpay. It is okay if they are being subsidized, but they—out of their own pocket, will say, you know what, thanks, but no thanks. Has this worked at all? Go ahead. I mean, if we are trying to get to an end here, what has it done?

Mr. MILLER. Well, I always try to be a little more balanced in this approach. We had a lot of bad policies incorporated into the Affordable Care Act, not the individual mandate alone. The way I would first put it is the individual mandate, not only did it not work, it didn't save those other bad policies. So we need to reexamine more than just the individual mandate itself.

The reason why coverage may not be attractive to people may be a part of the way in which we tried to standardize coverage in certain ways, which meant that suddenly it no longer appealed to people in the same manner when they were paying more of the cost than they did before and weren't highly subsidized. So we have got a lot of different things to take out of the bottle and reassemble. But the individual mandate itself did not provide some extra boost.

And you can't keep subsidizing people to basically say, come on. Instead, what we got were limited networks, lower actuarial values, and higher deductibles for people who saw the cost and they didn't want that coverage and they are complaining to you about it. That is how we created a new distortion to deal with the old distortions.

Mr. MCDONOUGH. Can I address?

Mr. KELLY. Oh, yes. Please. Sure.

Mr. MCDONOUGH. Thank you for the question. So just the question, does this work? Well, work is obviously in the eye of the beholder. But just let me give you some responses to does this law work.

Mr. KELLY. Can you do that, Mr. McDonough, if it is in the eye of the beholder? Yeah, I have got two or three pages of people back home in my district, they are saying it doesn't work. So in the eyes of a lot of beholders, including the majority of this country, it doesn't work.

Mr. MCDONOUGH. Okay. So lowest rate of uninsurance in the history of the United States. Drop the——

Mr. KELLY. But, sir, listen, I don't want to equate having an insurance policy with having health care. Huge difference.

Mr. MCDONOUGH. Rates of satisfaction among people who have been enrolled in Medicaid and people who have been enrolled in exchange policies, around 80 percent satisfaction. Drop in the rate of uninsurance among America's children, by 50 percent over the past several years. The rate of financial security and the drop in medical debt experienced by Americans across the country, a substantial drop. Rate of increase in per enrollee Medicare spending is the lowest it has been in the history of the program since it was created in 1965. Those are just five things. We can go on and on.

Mr. KELLY. Where is this study from?

Mr. MCDONOUGH. These are all different studies, sir. I would be happy to share the sources of all of those with you.

Mr. KELLY. Okay. I would like to see that information. And I appreciate that.

Mr. MCDONOUGH. Happy to do that.

Mr. KELLY. Mr. Graham.

Mr. GRAHAM. I think what Professor McDonough stated, those facts are certainly cohere with what I understand of a lot of things, but very little of that has to do with the individual mandate. You know, there has been some Medicare changes going on. Most of the effect of the Affordable Care Act in terms of coverage is Medicaid. And I know I am going to provoke some folks here, but I don't like to include Medicaid as insurance because Medicaid is a welfare program. So as long as we include more Medicaid enrollment as insured, that is like saying more TANF with having a job, it doesn't make any sense, you know.

So if we are going to be coherent or whatever, giving people more welfare benefits, that's fine. If that is what you all want to do, that is your prerogative as the folks who tax and spend, that's what you are going to do. But let's not pretend that we are making people more individually responsible through this mandate. And as you say, for very many people, the small business owner, the self-employed person, it is just driving them crazy, as we have heard from you and so many of your colleagues, trying to figure out what the heck is going on, how to get an affordable plan and——

Mr. KELLY. I know. We are going to continue to work, Chairman, and I appreciate, again, being included. We are going to continue to try to work to make sure that the American people understand. They are not going to lose, by the way, their insurance. I mean, Mr. Trump was sworn in last Friday. I don't think anybody is walking around the country right now and had their insurance pulled away from them, so that is kind of a false narrative. But we have got to find something that makes sense. None of this makes sense to me economically. Why would anybody stay in the insurance business to lose money?

Thank you.

Chairman BUCHANAN. I now recognize myself. We spent a lot of time on the mandate. I want to shift gears a little bit and talk about affordability and access.

My background before I got here, I have been here about 10 years, but before that, 30 years. And I think back 30, 40 years ago, companies paid or people had access to low cost, high quality health care. I thought back a few days ago and I was thinking back 20 years ago when I was chairman of the chamber in our area, we had 2,500 businesses, most of them 15 employees or less. The number one issue, 20 years ago—and this before the ACA to give them—you know, we can talk about that a little bit.

But 20 years ago, the number one issue, we surveyed all our members, was access and affordable health care. And it just seems like it has accelerated to the point of being absurd that typical individuals—it is not unusual in my area in Florida, Sarasota Florida, a couple could be paying $2,000 a month for health care. That is outrageous. That is more than a car payment and a house payment.

I read the other day, and I shared this with our people, in the front page of I think it was USA Today, 62 percent of Americans don't have $1,000 in the bank. I thought to myself when I looked back, you know, you can talk about wages and everything else, that one of the things that is gutting the middle class I think is health care cost. You get the subsidy. You know, maybe it works for you, but people just outside the subsidy, because small businesses and everybody else, they can't afford to provide it. It's $1,400 for a family of four, $1,600. So the small business might pick up $600,

$700. It is getting passed to the workers. And that is why nobody has anything.

So my thought when I first heard about the ACA, I was concerned back then about the cost of health care and I was open-minded, if it bent a curve on health care. But I heard what you said, Doctor. But I can just tell you in our region in Florida, it is not unusual to hear every single day rates going up 20 and 30 percent for small businesses and individuals. That is the reality.

So I guess I would ask any of you, Mr. Miller, Mr. Graham, let's start there, what are we going to do about, or your thoughts, in bending the curve? It is just—and I know it is a big discussion, but I would like to just have maybe 30 seconds each of you just to give me your point.

Mr. MILLER. All right. That is a bigger discussion.

Chairman BUCHANAN. I know it is a big discussion.

Mr. MILLER. So let me simplify. This may not be the politically astute answer.

Chairman BUCHANAN. No. I just want——

Mr. MILLER. If we keep pumping more money into health care, it is going to cost more. Now, if we want to do that, we need to think about that a little bit more surgically. So the approach might be to actually have the individuals supposedly benefiting from this to control those dollars and decide how they want to spend it. That will be a different type of result in terms of better quality health care at a lower price over time. We have tried subsidizing it, we have tried regulating it, we have tried placating everybody in between. We need to get it down to the ground level and decide what people actually want to spend their money on. And that includes trading off health care with better wages. And we need to stimulate economic growth and we need a healthier population. We need a better health care delivery system.

Those are all things well beyond the little games we play with individual mandates and insurance subsidies. That is a bigger discussion, but we need to focus more on that.

Mr. GRAHAM. I would agree with Mr. Miller. And I would point out that all this money going into the ObamaCare exchanges, it really goes to insurance companies, you know. We advocate consumer-driven health care. We don't give any tax credits to individuals that they can spend directly. And I know one of the Members talked about the premium is more than the rent. Well, when I pay my rent, I move in that day and I start living there, you know. I pay for these insurance policies and they don't kick in until I go to the hospital. So if we are going to help people, let's help them pay directly for care. And we had some good experience that that can help reduce some cost.

Chairman BUCHANAN. Doctor, I will give you an opportunity. Take a few seconds and wrap up.

Mr. MCDONOUGH. The major challenge, it seems to me and to many other experts with whom I work, is to change the underlying incentives in terms of the delivery of medical care to move away from a system that rewards providers to do more and more through fee-for-service and, instead, to move toward a system that rewards providers when they actually provide quality, value service. And we have a number of important directions that we are going in.

The Nation is moving in this direction, regardless of what happens to the fate of the ACA. You saw it in the MACRA law, the bipartisan bill that passed the House and the Senate in 2015. That is not a rejection of the direction that the ACA started, it is an enhancement and an acceleration of it. That is going to continue. And I think that is really probably the most important dynamic that is going on right now in terms of moving our system to a different place.

Chairman BUCHANAN. Let me just conclude. In Florida—I was chairman actually in the floor of the chamber down there too—it is the biggest issue. The cost of health care keeps going. It is not just the last 8 years. It has been the last 20 years. It is out of control, out of hand. We have got to find a way we can work together for the betterment of everybody in the country.

I would like to thank our witnesses for appearing before us today. Please be advised that Members have 2 weeks to submit written questions to be answered later in writing. Those questions and your answers will be part of the formal hearing record.

With that, the Subcommittee stands adjourned.
[Whereupon, at 3:45 p.m., the Subcommittee was adjourned.] [Public Submissions for the Record follows:]

STATEMENT ON "THE INDIVIDUAL MANDATE UNDER THE AFFORDABLE CARE ACT" SUBMITTED TO THE HOUSE WAYS AND MEANS COMMITTEE SUBCOMMITTEE ON OVERSIGHT

January 24, 2017

America's Health Insurance Plans (AHIP) is the national association whose members provide coverage for health care and related services. Through these offerings, we improve and protect the health and financial security of consumers, families, businesses, communities and the nation. We are committed to market-based solutions and public-private partnerships that improve affordability, value, access and well-being for consumers.

We appreciate this opportunity to comment on the individual mandate established by the Affordable Care Act (ACA). Our members have strongly supported an approach to health reform that brings everyone into the system. Broad coverage can ensure the availability of affordable coverage options. Health insurance only works when everyone is covered: those who utilize insurance to obtain quality care as well as those who are healthy but have insurance to protect them in case they get sick. Both types of consumers must be insured for coverage to remain affordable.

As the committee examines this issue, we recognize that the individual market has been a challenge for many years - both before the ACA and after. We recognize that certain parts of the ACA have not worked as well as intended, particularly for individuals who purchase coverage on their own. The challenges facing the individual exchange marketplace - which have been well-documented - include significant increases in average premiums in 2017, fewer health plan choices, and lower-than-expected exchange enrollment and risk pool stability challenges in some states. And absent significant and specific improvements to the exchanges this year, 2018 was already likely to be another challenging year.

While these challenges are real and remain, it is also true that the health reform law has expanded coverage to 20 million Americans. These gains have been achieved through Medicaid expansion as well as through the ACA exchange marketplaces (which has been accomplished through financial assistance via premium subsidies and through the individual mandate).

We also recognize that Congress is preparing to consider legislation to substantially change the ACA and that the individual mandate is likely to be repealed as part of this effort. That's why we are so focused on finding the right solutions that can deliver the strong, stable market - and affordable coverage - that we all want to achieve. We believe it is important for Congress to approve continuous coverage incentives - along with additional stabilization solutions - to minimize the impact of eliminating the individual mandate.

Our statement focuses on two topics:

- The rationale for having full consumer participation, in combination with market reforms and financial assistance, as part of a strategy for achieving a balanced risk pool in the individual health insurance market.
- The need for effective policies to encourage continuous coverage and broad consumer participation in the individual health insurance market if Congress passes legislation to repeal the ACA individual mandate and retains all other market reforms.

The Rationale for Full Consumer Participation

Since January 2014, the ACA has required health plans to offer coverage to everyone, including individuals with pre-existing conditions, and has prohibited any variation in premiums based on a person's health status or medical history. The health reform law also requires everyone to purchase and maintain coverage (or else pay a penalty) in recognition of the fact that, without such a requirement, there otherwise would be a strong incentive for people to wait and purchase insurance only after they get sick or injured.

In 2012, while the U.S. Supreme Court was weighing its decision about the constitutionality of the individual mandate and other ACA provisions, we commissioned studies examining the experience of two states - Washington and Kentucky-that enacted market reforms without an individual mandate or any other mechanism to achieve universal access to coverage. These studies yielded important lessons about the unintended consequences of health reforms that create incentives for healthy people to forego the purchase of coverage:

- One study[51] examined Washington state's experiment with guarantee issue in the absence of an individual mandate. According to the study, the reforms Washington state enacted in 1993 resulted in substantial increases in the premiums charged for individually purchased policies, a dramatic reduction in the number of carriers writing policies for individuals in the state, and a 30 percent increase in the number of uninsured.
- Another study[52] explained that the enactment of guarantee issue and community rating reforms in Kentucky, in the absence of an individual mandate, provided a powerful incentive for people to delay purchasing coverage until after they needed medical care. As a result of these reforms, individuals' insurance premiums skyrocketed, in some cases over 100 percent, and the resulting

---

[51] Lessons Learned: Washington State's 1993 Experiment with Health Insurance Reforms, May 2012.
[52] Unintended Consequences: Kentucky's Experiment with Health Care Offers Lessons For Nation, May 2012.

disruption in the state's insurance marketplace forced most of the state's health insurers to leave the market.

In addition to experience in the states, several non-partisan studies have concluded that eliminating the individual mandate would significantly increase premiums and cause serious market disruptions, absent the implementation of additional or alternative policies to promote market stability.

- The Congressional Budget Office (CBO) concluded that "premiums in the non-group market would be roughly 20 percent to 25 percent higher than under current law" as a result of "repealing the penalties associated with the individual mandate."[53] However, CBO's analysis did not evaluate the impact of any alternatives to the individual mandate that policymakers may consider.
- The American Academy of Actuaries has cautioned that "eliminating the ACA's individual mandate, premium subsidies or cost-sharing reductions would increase the likelihood for adverse selection, in which people who are most at risk of high health care costs would be the most likely to enroll, while many healthier individuals decide not to purchase coverage. Premiums for the remaining pool would increase as a result, further exacerbating adverse selection problems. A premium spiral could result, with fewer and fewer insureds and higher and higher premiums.[54]
- The Brookings Institution cautioned that eliminating the individual mandate penalties "would likely de-stabilize the market and very possibly cause it to collapse in some regions of the country during the interim period before any replacement is designed." Moreover,

---

[53] Congressional Budget Office. "How Repealing Certain Portions of the ACA Would Affect Health Insurance Coverage and Premiums." January 2017. https://www.cbogov/sites/default/files/115th-congress-20172018/reports/52371-coverageandpremiums.pdf.

[54] American Academy of Actuaries. "Consequences of Repealing ACA Provisions or Ending Cost-Sharing Reduction Reimbursements." December 7, 2016. http://actuary.org/files/publications/HPC_letter_ACACSR_120716.pdf.

the Brookings authors found that eliminating the mandate penalties would **cause a substantial number of those currently with insurance, especially younger, heathier ones, to drop their insurance, leaving an even sicker pool in place and increasing premiums even further."[55]

These research findings are well worth considering in the congressional debate on ACA replacement reforms. The clear lesson for policymakers is that any reforms that give healthy people incentives to delay purchasing coverage will lead to unintended consequences—higher costs and fewer choices for the broader population. It will diminish access to high quality, affordable health insurance. To avoid this outcome, Congress should take steps to encourage continuous coverage and broad participation in the individual health insurance market.

Alternative Approaches to Encouraging Continuous Coverage and Broad Participation in the Individual Health Insurance Market

We recognize there is significant support in Congress for repealing the individual mandate penalties, as part of a broader ACA repeal bill. However, absent the enactment of alternative incentives to promote continuous coverage, this could create market instability and result in the loss of health insurance coverage for millions of Americans.

To promote a stable individual market during a transition period, incentives are needed to encourage consumers to maintain continuous coverage and minimize movement in and out of the marketplace. We have developed a potential framework of public policies to implement effective continuous coverage requirements, leveraging existing statutes and current health plan practices.

---

[55] Brookings Institution. "Why Repealing the ACA before Replacing it Won't Work and What Might." December 13, 2016. https://www.brookings.edu/research/why-repealing-the-aca-before-replacing-it-wont-work-and-whatmight/.

A framework for continuous coverage must begin with a clear definition of requirements, which must be clearly communicated to consumers. We recommend using the existing HIPAA framework as the starting point to define continuous coverage. While HIPAA requires 18 months of creditable medical coverage, we recommend the requirement be set at 12 months as this better reflects coverage trends in the individual market. Creditable coverage should leverage the existing definition of minimum essential coverage (MEC) - a well-defined, existing standard.

Once new rules of the road are in place, all consumers should have the opportunity to enroll in coverage during 2018 open enrollment, regardless of their current coverage status, before any new requirements are put in place. Education and awareness are critical to ensure consumers understand the consequences of waiting to enroll, and these new requirements should be clearly communicated to enrollees during 2017 to encourage enrollment during 2018 open enrollment.

Individuals who apply for coverage after January 31, 2018 (after the close of the 2018 open enrollment period) must meet continuous coverage requirements, defined as 12 months of creditable coverage. Those who do not meet this requirement would face penalties such as a premium surcharge or having to wait six months to enroll similar to the existing practice for Medicare Parts B and D.

Other policy requirements need to be implemented in tandem to promote continuous coverage and reduce movement in and out of the individual market risk pool. Individual market special enrollment period (SEP) rules should be modified, as appropriate, to reflect continuous coverage policies. SEP rules should be tightened so that a life event is not an opportunity to enroll in coverage for the first time, but to make a needed change to an existing policy (e.g., to add a newborn). SEP rules must be enforced and eligibility should be verified prior to enrollment.

Implementing effective and well-designed continuous coverage incentives is critical to promoting affordable coverage and market stability-especially if the individual mandate is eliminated immediately under partial repeal of the ACA through a budget reconciliation bill. In addition to continuous coverage incentives, additional policies such as risk pool funding, reforms to the premium subsidies (APTC) and related policies are necessary to mitigate coverage disruptions and can help promote a more stable transition to alternative insurance coverage reforms.

Conclusion

Policymakers in Washington and in state capitols across the country have tried to improve the individual insurance market for many years. This is another opportunity to get it right. And by working together to find the most effective solutions, we can deliver the long-term improvements that the American people deserve.

INDEX

A

ABA, 85
access, 30, 32, 41, 72, 117, 133, 134, 143, 145, 147, 150, 157, 160, 183, 191, 194, 206, 230, 270, 274, 275, 285, 289, 293
accessibility, 157
accommodation, 211
accountability, 188
accounting, 74, 75
acquisitions, 10, 12, 15, 17, 22, 24, 28, 31, 39, 42, 50, 56, 69, 70, 72, 74, 84, 118, 124, 127, 139, 144, 146, 149, 150, 167, 168, 175, 193, 196
adjustment, 255, 256
adults, 236, 277
advocacy, 87, 88, 244
Affordable Care Act, ix, 72, 83, 136, 168, 174, 185, 209, 210, 212, 213, 217, 219, 220, 221, 222, 226, 228, 229, 230, 233, 239, 242, 244, 247, 250, 258, 260, 262, 263, 267, 268, 275, 277, 282, 284, 288, 289
agencies, 38, 48, 50, 65, 68, 81, 84, 85, 86, 90, 135, 149
agriculture, 34

airline industry, 75
Alaska, 87, 256, 268
Alphabet, 111
American workers, 3, 6
annual rate, 56, 168
antitrust, 4, 7, 29, 32, 38, 48, 50, 63, 69, 84, 85, 87, 88, 90, 131, 146, 149, 151, 152, 171
appendectomy, 137
architect, 178
arthroscopy, 190, 193
aspiration, 111, 112
assessment, 87, 92, 97, 105, 106, 204, 254
assets, 85, 159, 169, 232, 253
attachment, 101
Attorney General, 88
audit, 112, 124
audits, 187
authorities, 85, 130, 133, 151, 152, 153, 176
authority, 121, 151
awareness, 294

B

bargaining, 41, 56, 64, 67, 68, 82, 120, 127, 159, 204

barriers, 44, 105, 108, 206
barriers to entry, 44, 206
base, 158, 159
behavioral change, 266
bending, 286
beneficiaries, 55, 56, 80, 176, 185, 190, 191, 193, 194, 197, 221, 224, 278
benefits, 5, 8, 21, 22, 24, 34, 36, 45, 47, 54, 63, 65, 67, 68, 69, 81, 87, 101, 118, 141, 160, 171, 222, 232, 239, 241, 254, 284
bias, 181
birth control, 145
births, 143
blind spot, 219
blood, 272
break-even, 256
brothers, 269, 271
Bureau of Labor Statistics, 56
burn, 138
Bush, President George Walker, 251
business costs, 264
business model, 92, 94, 95, 96, 97, 98, 99, 100, 101, 111, 112, 156
business processes, 93, 99
business strategy, 94, 99
businesses, 134, 154, 285, 288
buyers, 83, 89

C

cancer, 171, 174
cancer care, 171
candidates, 105, 109, 252
cardiac surgery, 51
cardiologist, 197
care model, 93, 96, 99, 147
case studies, 143
case study, 54, 57, 58
cash, 220, 225, 264
cash flow, 220, 264
catalyst, 100

categorization, 106, 117
CDC, 254
Census, 38, 58
certificate, 47, 69, 86, 87, 130, 143
chain of production, 71
challenges, 86, 87, 88, 110, 152, 176, 259, 265, 289
chaos, 92
chemotherapy, 172
Chicago, 49, 55, 158
Chief Justice, 236
children, 155, 214, 283
cities, 76
citizens, 218, 236, 255, 257, 264
clarity, 112
Clayton Act, 85, 151
clients, 211, 249
Clinton Administration, 250
Clinton, Senator Hillary, 252
closure, 276
clothing, 37
coercion, 234, 260
collaboration, 50
color, v, 145, 147
commerce, 87, 236
commercial, 5, 8, 39, 57, 64, 68, 74, 75, 81, 90, 92, 97, 127, 131, 134, 164, 170, 186, 197
commodity, 36, 181
communities, 10, 12, 131, 145, 146, 163, 183, 288
community, 16, 19, 132, 147, 155, 173, 183, 186, 239, 276, 291
compensation, 37, 49, 56, 113, 118, 180, 181
competition, ix, 5, 8, 9, 10, 13, 15, 21, 23, 27, 29, 31, 32, 33, 34, 35, 37, 38, 41, 42, 43, 44, 45, 46, 47, 48, 49, 50, 51, 53, 54, 55, 58, 62, 63, 66, 67, 68, 73, 74, 75, 76, 81, 82, 85, 87, 89, 118, 129, 137, 142, 148, 149, 150, 151, 153, 154, 155, 157,

160, 165,167, 172, 173, 174, 175, 176, 177, 185, 195, 199, 203, 212, 273
competitive markets, 64, 151
competitiveness, 199
competitors, 10, 12, 29, 31, 32, 33, 34, 38, 41, 42, 44, 46, 117, 118, 129, 158
complexity, 138, 194, 274
compliance, 157, 210, 211, 227, 228, 233, 235, 237, 240, 265, 266
composition, 183
compression, 266
conflict, 186, 231
conflict of interest, 186
congress, 292
Congress, vi, 1, 2, 5, 9, 14, 16, 18, 20, 64, 65, 68, 89, 123, 124, 131, 133, 155, 156, 164, 165, 170, 172, 173, 174, 176, 179, 188, 197, 198, 200, 221, 236, 238, 250, 254, 255, 256, 275, 276, 289, 290, 293
Congressional Budget Office, 63, 66, 216, 217, 222, 228, 235, 249, 250, 292
consensus, 248
consent, 19, 20, 25, 84, 105, 129
consolidation, 3, 4, 5, 6, 7, 8, 9, 11, 12, 13, 15, 16, 17, 18, 19, 20, 21, 22, 23, 24, 25, 27, 28, 29, 30, 31, 32, 34, 36, 37, 38, 39, 40, 41, 43, 44, 45, 46, 47, 50, 51, 54, 56, 58, 62, 63, 64, 65, 66, 67, 68, 69, 70, 71, 72, 73, 74, 76, 77, 78, 80, 81, 83, 84, 85, 86, 87, 88, 89, 90, 91, 94, 96, 117, 118, 119, 120, 121, 126, 128, 129, 134, 135, 139, 140, 141, 145, 146, 147, 148, 149, 153, 155, 156, 157, 159, 160, 161, 164, 165, 166, 167, 169, 170, 171, 172, 173, 174, 175, 177, 178, 183, 184, 185, 191, 193, 195, 200,202, 203
constituents, 131, 213, 273, 274, 282
Constitution, 236
consulting, 107
consumer choice, 183, 186, 187, 188
consumers, 4, 7, 9, 10, 11, 12, 13, 15, 17, 18, 19, 20, 21, 22, 23, 24, 25, 30, 32, 36, 37, 40, 48, 63, 65, 67, 69, 75, 77, 83, 85, 89, 90, 94, 96, 100, 101, 120, 121, 122, 125, 128, 134, 135, 140, 141, 146, 156, 177, 183, 186, 187, 188, 205, 206, 239, 243, 245, 246, 248, 253, 257, 258, 278, 288, 289, 294
controversial, 180, 256, 259
controversies, 256
conversations, 255
cooperative agreements, 87
coordination, 10, 12, 15, 18, 28, 45, 46, 81, 83, 118, 169
cosmetic, 179
cost, 3, 14, 15, 17, 18, 28, 34, 42, 46, 64, 67, 69, 79, 80, 82, 88, 91, 94, 96, 100, 117, 119, 123, 124, 128, 130, 131, 133, 140, 142, 161, 163, 164, 170, 171, 173, 182, 187, 188, 190, 191, 192, 193, 194, 197, 204, 225, 228, 233, 237, 241, 246, 248, 249, 251,257, 258, 259, 260, 261, 271, 275, 277, 280, 282, 283, 285, 286, 287, 288, 292
cost saving, 64, 67, 119, 140
costs of compliance, 232
costs of production, 205
counsel, 25, 26
covering, 184
creativity, 110
crowding out, 36
CSR, 248
culture, 91, 95, 97, 108, 111
customers, 41, 70, 129, 206, 229, 241

D

damages, v
danger, 249
data collection, 105
data set, 105, 269
database, 64, 68, 90, 105, 150, 152
deaths, 44

defendants, 49
demand curve, 204
Democrat, 251
Department of Commerce, 58
Department of Defense, 163
Department of Health and Human Services, 21, 24, 76
Department of Justice, 4, 7, 21, 23, 38, 53, 85, 151, 160, 176
destruction, 94, 100
Diabetes, 10, 13
dialysis, 77
differentiated products, 176
diffusion, 114
directors, 109
discharges, 3, 6
disclosure, 155
distortions, 29, 32, 283
distribution, 109
district courts, 85
District of Columbia, 249
diversity, 147
DOC, 154
doctors, 3, 6, 35, 39, 118, 136, 138, 147, 148, 149, 182, 191, 194, 272, 273, 274
DOJ, 4, 7, 73, 176, 177
dominance, 191, 195, 200, 202, 203
draft, 99
drinking water, 180
drugs, 10, 13, 155, 173, 184
dynamism, 27, 31, 35, 47

E

earnings, 184
economic activity, 275
economic growth, 287
economic integration, 50
economic theory, 204
economics, 25, 27, 204, 215, 218, 219, 277
economies of scale, 82, 169

ecosystem, 111
editors, 51, 52, 53, 54, 55
e-mail, 189, 199, 201
emergency, 51, 137, 216, 220, 224, 225, 266, 275
employee compensation, 49
employees, 16, 18, 41, 65, 68, 89, 90, 108, 109, 121, 122, 285
employers, 11, 13, 29, 32, 36, 40, 41, 43, 48, 65, 68, 74, 76, 89, 90, 118, 121, 122, 123, 152, 156, 231
employment, 74, 80, 93, 99, 113, 125, 190, 193, 196, 226, 232
employment status, 232
energy, 110
enforcement, 29, 32, 38, 48, 65, 68, 69, 84, 85, 86, 90, 130, 146, 151, 152, 153, 160, 232, 233, 237, 240, 265
enrollment, 54, 175, 229, 233, 238, 239, 240, 241, 243, 245, 247, 252, 253, 255, 256, 265, 266, 276, 279, 280, 281, 284, 289, 294, 295
enrollment rates, 239
entrepreneurs, 51, 108
environment, 102, 111, 112, 131, 262, 265
equilibrium, 204
equipment, 70, 162, 191, 195, 200, 202, 203
evidence, 22, 24, 29, 31, 33, 34, 35, 38, 40, 41, 42, 43, 45, 46, 51, 52, 56, 63, 64, 67, 68, 73, 75, 76, 77, 78, 81, 82, 83, 87, 93, 96, 98, 99, 100, 110, 117, 118, 121, 126, 127, 128, 135, 136, 139, 140, 143, 153, 158, 159, 171, 186, 193, 195, 219, 225, 226, 243, 245, 247, 255, 279
evidence-based practices, 110
evolution, 240
exclusion, 211
execution, 110
Executive Order, 8, 165
exercise, 83, 185, 204, 236, 237
exercises, 205

expenditures, 9, 10, 12, 22, 24, 46, 57, 71, 98, 162, 163, 197, 276
expertise, 65, 68, 88, 90, 121, 154, 175, 239
externalities, 204

F

faculty positions, 66
faith, 252
families, 3, 6, 36, 155, 213, 253, 257, 259, 264, 288
farmers, 264
FDA, 129, 185
federal courts, 176
federal government, 188, 218, 223, 225, 259, 271
federal law, 178, 187
Federal Trade Commission (FTC), 4, 7, 27, 33, 38, 53, 55, 63, 66, 73, 84, 86, 87, 121, 129, 131, 143, 149, 150, 151, 152, 153, 156, 157, 158, 159, 160, 165, 167, 168, 176, 184, 195, 196, 197, 204
Federal Trade Commission Act, 121
fertilization, 145
financial, 4, 8, 28, 57, 64, 65, 68, 89, 90, 92, 95, 98, 103, 106, 107, 108, 109, 116, 117, 130, 134, 136, 171, 172, 197, 255, 257, 263, 276, 283, 288, 289, 290
financial incentives, 28, 65, 68, 90
financial performance, 95
fiscal year, 269
food, 34, 37
force, 110, 127, 187, 227, 228, 231, 238
foreign nationals, 233
formula, 179, 186, 242, 245, 248, 249, 258
forward integration, 89
foundations, 228, 238
freedom, 236, 252
fringe benefits, 37
funding, 112, 266, 295
funds, 65, 67, 68, 81, 90, 109, 222, 227, 231

G

GAO, 22, 168, 172, 173, 174
GDP, 34, 72, 162
general practitioner, 73
general surgeon, 182
Georgia, 154, 157
good deed, 123
goods and services, 36
Google, 111, 115
government spending, 216, 219, 226
governments, 48
governor, 268
grants, 90
graph, 281
Great Recession, 226
gross domestic product, 2, 6, 162
grouping, 77
growth, 22, 24, 54, 56, 75, 77, 88, 168, 174, 216, 219, 225, 228, 238, 256, 267, 268
growth rate, 168
guidelines, 53, 153, 211

H

hair, 148
harmful effects, 126
Health and Human Services, 5, 8, 162, 163 230, 292
health care professionals, 77
health care sector, 32, 35, 70, 71, 87, 161
health care system, 31, 32, 35, 102, 104, 110, 111, 188, 216, 227, 231
health condition, 145, 230
health expenditure, 133, 163
health insurance, 4, 7, 33, 34, 36, 39, 42, 44, 49, 51, 52, 69, 75, 83, 101, 118, 121, 134, 150, 157, 159, 163, 174, 177, 179, 213, 219, 220, 226, 232, 233, 234, 236, 237, 239, 241, 242, 243, 245, 246, 247, 248, 250, 251, 252, 253, 254, 255, 256,

257, 260, 262, 263, 264, 265, 267, 268, 272, 275, 278, 279, 290, 293, 294
health services, 147, 226
health status, 229, 240, 246, 290
healthcare consolidation, vii, 1, 2, 6
healthcare costs, 4, 7, 11, 13, 14, 15, 17, 18, 30, 50, 87, 92, 94, 118, 122, 133
healthcare spending, 2, 6, 133
heart attack, 43, 44
hematology, 17, 19, 81, 173
HHS, ix, 5, 8, 9, 212, 215, 256
history, 166, 219, 238, 263, 273, 281, 283, 284
homes, 275
horizontal integration, 167, 206
horizontal merger, 4, 7, 49, 63, 67, 73, 126, 151, 160, 176
hospital consolidation, 3, 5, 6, 8, 17, 19, 41, 50, 54, 58, 73, 91, 96, 139, 140, 170, 173
host, 82, 87, 153
House, 1, 25, 30, 57, 66, 161, 165, 183, 184, 185, 189, 192, 198, 199, 200, 201, 209, 210, 229, 244, 249, 251, 253, 278, 287, 288
House of Representatives, 1, 30, 161, 165, 183, 189, 192, 198, 200, 244, 251, 253
household income, 234
housing, 37
HPC, 88, 134, 135, 248, 292
human, 122, 214, 277
human resources, 122
human right, 214
hunting, 269

I

identification, 52
image, 234
imbalances, 232
immigrants, 233
improvements, 37, 158, 226, 234, 289, 295

incidence, 50, 54
income, 216, 220, 228, 231, 232, 233, 234, 235, 237, 239, 246, 257, 258, 259, 265, 266, 273, 274, 280
income tax, 233, 234, 235, 265
incubator, 107
individuals, ix, 33, 35, 36, 82, 93, 98, 102, 104, 106, 134, 183, 212, 220, 221, 228, 229, 231, 233, 235, 237, 240, 250, 253, 254, 257, 260, 263, 264, 265, 267, 274, 280, 285, 286, 287, 289, 290, 291, 292
industrial organization, 52, 53
industries, 40, 70
industry, 3, 4, 5, 6, 7, 8, 15, 16, 17, 18, 20, 23, 34, 37, 39, 52, 54, 56, 62, 63, 64, 65, 66, 67, 68, 70, 72, 73, 81, 84, 86, 87, 89, 90, 105, 114, 117, 118, 139, 148, 159, 164, 165, 166, 167, 174, 183, 186, 187, 191, 195, 200, 202, 203, 247, 254, 257, 268
industry consolidation, 52, 62, 64, 66, 68, 84, 90, 148
inequality, 56
infancy, 113, 122, 135
inflation, 233, 257
information technology, 99
informed consent, 234
infrastructure, 48
injury, v, 214, 265
institutions, 69, 84, 108, 276
insulin, 10, 13, 120
insurance policy, 283
integration, 45, 46, 49, 50, 56, 57, 79, 140, 141, 148, 156, 167, 196, 197, 205
intermediaries, 86
internal controls, 95
Internal Revenue Service, 216, 228, 232
internists, 73
interoperability, 199
investment, 37, 64, 68, 92, 98, 108, 109, 112, 163
investments, 28, 45, 92, 93, 94, 98, 99

investors, 74, 184
IRS, 221, 234, 235, 254, 274
issues, 5, 8, 10, 11, 13, 14, 20, 22, 23, 25, 112, 120, 132, 133, 140, 143, 148, 151, 153, 157, 160, 177, 180, 236, 267, 274

J

Joint Economic Committee, 230
judiciary, 174, 175, 185
Judiciary Committee, 129, 184
jurisdiction, 156

K

Kennedy, Edward Moore, 251
Kennedy, John Fitzgerald, 62, 65
kicks, 178

L

labor market, 49, 51
landscape, 15, 17, 55, 151, 174
laws, 4, 7, 47, 69, 87, 132, 151, 171, 187, 246
lawyers, 137
lead, 4, 7, 15, 18, 22, 24, 29, 31, 37, 38, 41, 43, 44, 87, 95, 112, 117, 118, 121, 137, 139, 148, 152, 164, 187, 247, 253, 293
leadership, 14, 91, 93, 95, 97, 98, 103, 104, 108, 268
learning, 5, 8, 99, 213, 238, 269
legislation, 47, 49, 84, 250, 251, 252, 253, 254, 278, 289, 290
legs, 246
lens, 92, 97, 154, 192, 196, 200, 202, 205, 206
lifetime, 240, 254
light, 110, 277
Likert scale, 105

Louisiana, 250
love, 120, 130, 263, 282
lower prices, 21, 23, 34, 36

M

magnitude, 93
majority, 3, 5, 6, 8, 35, 38, 42, 74, 93, 98, 107, 121, 148, 163, 224, 236, 275, 283
management, 74, 88, 123, 169, 177
mania, 167
manufacturing, 34, 167, 204
manufacturing companies, 167
marginal product, 205
marginalization, 205
market concentration, 38, 39, 45, 53, 77, 126, 164, 174, 184
market position, 28, 203
market share, 4, 7, 28, 38, 39, 44, 51, 70, 75, 80, 155, 174, 185, 191, 195, 200, 202, 203
market structure, 49, 55
marketing, 206
marketplace, 43, 129, 137, 183, 184, 185, 187, 188, 203, 213, 255, 256, 263, 272, 275, 276, 289, 292, 294
mass, 203, 224
materials, 211, 212
matter, v, 35, 259, 277
media, 149, 174, 175
median, 93, 98, 103, 108, 109, 116, 117
Medicaid, 47, 64, 67, 71, 72, 101, 133, 138, 145, 150, 162, 163, 181, 182, 217, 219, 222, 223, 224, 225, 228, 238, 239, 247, 266, 269, 270, 274, 275, 276, 277, 280, 281, 282, 283, 284, 289
medical, 34, 42, 65, 69, 70, 98, 132, 138, 149, 162, 171, 180, 181, 182, 203, 219, 234, 242, 245, 246, 249, 253, 254, 255, 262, 263, 264, 272, 275, 276, 284, 287, 290, 291, 294

medical care, 69, 182, 287, 291
medical history, 219, 246, 262, 264, 290
Medicare, 3, 4, 5, 6, 8, 9, 12, 22, 24, 43, 44, 46, 47, 53, 55, 56, 64, 67, 71, 72, 75, 76, 80, 83, 99, 123, 124, 125, 127, 128, 133, 138, 150, 159, 162, 163, 164, 165, 168, 169, 170, 171, 172, 173, 174, 175, 176, 185, 190, 191, 193, 194, 196, 197, 219, 222, 240, 253, 275, 277, 284, 294
medication, 186
medicine, 25, 73, 109, 179, 182, 214
MedPAC, 3, 5, 6, 8, 164, 165, 170, 171, 173, 175, 176
memory, 153
mental health, 132
mergers, 4, 7, 9, 10, 12, 13, 15, 18, 21, 22, 23, 24, 27, 29, 31, 33, 38, 40, 41, 44, 49, 50, 52, 54, 57, 58, 67, 69, 70, 72, 73, 78, 79, 81, 82, 84, 86, 88, 89, 91, 92, 98, 126, 128, 129, 140, 141, 142, 143, 144, 145, 147, 149, 150, 151, 152, 158, 160, 166, 167,168, 175, 176, 177, 184
methodology, 105
metropolitan areas, 3, 6
Miami, 276
middle class, 36, 265, 285
migration, 94, 96, 101, 190, 191, 192, 193
miscarriages, 145
mission, 64, 67, 81, 104, 155, 214, 280
Missouri, 264, 265, 267
models, 82, 83, 92, 93, 97, 98, 99, 103, 111, 112, 113, 132, 197, 279, 281
modifications, 238
mole, 124
monopoly, 33, 85, 130, 204, 205
monopoly power, 205
monopsony, 83
moratorium, 137
mortality, 43, 44, 45, 73
mortality rate, 45
mosaic, 266
motivation, 82, 127

MRI, 134
myocardial infarction, 44

N

National Health Service, 44, 53
national mandate, 250
National Survey, 99, 101
negative consequences, 259
negotiating, 47, 67, 127, 131, 141, 152, 184, 206
negotiation, 82
neuroscience, 19
neutral, 125, 173
New England, 16, 19, 51, 81, 173, 239
NHS, 44, 51
normal profits, 204
nurses, 137
nursing, 132, 163
nursing care, 163
nursing home, 132

O

Obama Administration, 265, 279
Obama, President Barack, 219, 245, 250, 252, 254, 272, 273
obesity, 50
officials, 88
operations, 179, 275
opportunities, 104, 232
opt out, 241
organize, 179
outpatient, 22, 24, 66, 72, 80, 138, 168, 172, 173, 179, 182, 190, 191, 192, 193, 194
outreach, 106
overlap, 76, 77, 78
oversight, 19, 124, 213
ownership, 19, 46, 49, 55, 64, 67, 68, 70, 83, 88, 89, 134, 136, 142, 180, 186, 193, 196

P

parents, 155, 214
participants, 70, 71, 75, 106, 107, 108, 110, 129, 137, 141, 142, 149, 185, 260
patient care, 145, 161, 182
penalties, 26, 220, 221, 222, 227, 229, 232, 233, 235, 237, 239, 240, 243, 245, 249, 252, 255, 257, 292, 293, 294
percentile, 45
permission, v
permit, 189, 198, 201
personal choice, 236
personal responsibility, 213
persons with disabilities, 211
pharmaceutical, 3, 6, 15, 18, 63, 65, 66, 67, 68, 77, 153, 156, 165, 166
pharmaceuticals, 278
physicians, 3, 5, 7, 8, 10, 12, 28, 29, 31, 34, 39, 40, 45, 50, 52, 55, 57, 61, 74, 75, 79, 80, 83, 85, 120, 127, 136, 138, 141, 165, 166, 168, 169, 171, 172, 182, 191, 193, 194, 196, 197, 234
pitch, 270
playing, 124, 185
pleasure, 120
PM, 205, 210
polar, 204
policy, 15, 25, 29, 42, 53, 56, 88, 92, 97, 103, 111, 112, 124, 131, 164, 172, 173, 180, 197, 214, 218, 227, 228, 230, 235, 238, 239, 240, 241, 243, 244, 247, 248, 250, 252, 262, 265, 272, 282, 295
policy makers, 29
policy options, 56, 241
policy responses, 42, 53
policymakers, 32, 48, 292, 293
political leaders, 257
political power, 225
politics, 184, 215, 218, 227, 230
pools, 254, 279

popular support, 231
population, 74, 141, 142, 143, 147, 148, 164, 182, 248, 265, 270, 275, 277, 278, 279, 280, 287, 293
poverty, 243, 280
precedents, 85, 152
predictive accuracy, 235
premium costs, ix, 212, 234
preparation, v, 102, 105, 113
prescription drugs, 10, 13, 65, 68, 70, 90, 120, 162
president, 106, 276
President, 155, 215, 219, 245, 249, 250, 251, 252, 254, 269, 272, 273
price competition, 129
price effect, 52, 54, 57
price taker, 204
primary data, 150
primary function, 116
principles, 57, 155, 214, 227, 236
private sector, 88, 218
probability, 43, 232
producers, 192, 196, 200, 202, 205
production costs, 205
professionals, 196
profit, 16, 18, 58, 63, 66, 92, 97, 158, 184, 205
project, 33, 108, 153, 235
propaganda, 20
protection, 215, 228, 240, 253
public administration, 244
public health, 76, 244
public interest, 68, 121
public policy, 15, 27, 218
public-private partnerships, 289
punishment, 219
pure monopoly, 204

Q

quality control, 105

quality improvement, 73, 94, 100
quality of life, 35
questioning, 11, 281

R

radar, 15, 18
real numbers, 281
reality, 46, 150, 216, 258, 273, 278, 279, 282, 286
recall, 153, 180
recession, 226
recognition, 103, 110, 139, 290
recommendations, v, 14, 89
reconciliation, 295
recovery, 181, 242
reform, 33, 35, 44, 51, 53, 103, 113, 125, 140, 168, 173, 184, 185, 215, 219, 224, 225, 226, 244, 246, 249, 250, 251, 257, 258, 263, 278, 279, 290, 291, 293, 295
regulations, 47, 86, 187, 239, 240
regulatory bodies, 88
regulatory controls, 138
regulatory requirements, 65, 68, 90
reimburse, 137
reinsurance, 256, 268
rejection, 287
rent, 265, 278, 287
requirement(s), 149, 186, 187, 210, 211, 242, 243, 244, 245, 248, 252, 263, 267, 290, 294, 295
researchers, 43, 72, 75, 77, 83, 90, 139, 159, 171, 269
Residential, 70
resistance, 47
resource allocation, 104, 112
resources, 10, 12, 49, 55, 57, 87, 90, 102, 105, 153, 231
response, 5, 8, 84, 89, 102, 106, 108, 110, 112, 122, 134, 179, 204, 211, 228, 232, 238

restrictions, 145
restructuring, 56, 111
retail, 154, 155, 186, 203, 204, 205, 206
retirement, 163
revenue, 28, 102, 105, 125, 143, 166, 167, 174, 185, 217, 222, 228, 232, 235, 280
rewards, 63, 64, 67, 81, 84, 159, 194, 287
rhetoric, 46, 138
rights, v
risk, 28, 43, 44, 45, 86, 136, 141, 160, 214, 219, 220, 229, 237, 240, 242, 245, 246, 247, 248, 254, 256, 262, 279, 289, 290, 292, 295
risk profile, 248
risks, 228, 239
roots, 243
rules, 25, 64, 67, 128, 236, 249, 294, 295
rural areas, 132, 136, 150
rural counties, 143

S

safety, 73, 125, 279
savings, 10, 12, 83, 160, 186, 187
scale economies, 64, 67, 68, 81, 82
school, 138, 275, 276
science, 149, 232
scope, 47, 82, 85, 89, 151, 170, 227, 234, 258, 266
security, 259, 284, 288
self-assessment, 113
self-employed, 260, 284
seller(s), 82, 135
Senate, 87, 174, 175, 242, 244, 249, 251, 287
Senate Committee on the Judiciary, 174, 175
sensitivity, 88
service provider, 92
services, v, 4, 5, 7, 8, 10, 12, 22, 24, 28, 31, 34, 35, 37, 48, 64, 68, 72, 74, 79, 80, 85,

87, 88, 89, 90, 92, 94, 95, 96, 97, 98, 100, 101, 110, 118, 123, 125, 127, 133, 142, 143, 144, 145, 146, 147, 162, 165, 167, 169, 170, 171, 172, 176, 184, 190, 193, 204, 226, 234, 262, 277, 288
settlements, 84
shape, 56, 227, 228, 236, 238
shock, 231
shortfall, 94, 100
showing, 277
silver, 43
skimming, 137
small business, 264, 284, 286
small businesses, 286
small group insurance, ix, 212
solution, 50, 268, 278
specifications, 104
speech, 176
spending, 2, 6, 33, 34, 36, 42, 49, 50, 51, 54, 55, 56, 63, 67, 80, 81, 88, 118, 125, 133, 141, 162, 163, 164, 168, 194, 196, 222, 223, 224, 227, 231, 284
spillover effects, 125
stability, 4, 8, 238, 267, 289, 292, 295
stabilization, 263, 290
staffing, 112
stakeholders, 63, 67, 81, 88, 165, 167, 172
standard of living, 118
standardization, 105
state, 40, 42, 44, 47, 48, 67, 69, 78, 84, 86, 88, 126, 172, 187, 223, 224, 227, 236, 245, 249, 254, 255, 256, 257, 273, 291, 295
state authorities, 86
states, 42, 47, 74, 78, 248, 252, 257, 289, 291, 292
statistics, 71, 101, 106, 204, 213, 277
statutes, 85, 86, 90, 245, 294
structural changes, 70
structure, 70, 102, 103, 104, 105, 107, 108, 110, 111, 112, 138, 246, 255, 274
structuring, 251

Subsidies, 222, 239
subsidy, 228, 239, 280, 286
substitutes, 40
Sun, 74
supervision, 48
suppliers, 86
supply chain, 11, 13, 14, 17, 183, 191, 195, 200, 202, 203
Supreme Court, 236, 281, 291
surgical intervention, 65, 69
survival, 43, 227, 237
symptoms, 100

T

talent, 108
target, 78, 128, 228, 232, 259, 280, 281
target population, 232, 280, 281
tax credits, 220, 221, 225, 287
taxes, 227, 231, 232, 233
taxpayers, 9, 12, 218, 220, 221, 222, 223, 231, 232
technology, 94, 99, 100, 107, 108, 110, 111, 144
technology transfer, 108
telephone, 102, 211
territory, 75
thinning, 272
thoughts, 11, 13, 47, 122, 135, 179, 183, 286
time periods, 40
tobacco, 34
tooth, 269
trade, 38, 87, 204
training, 155, 273
trajectory, 109
transactions, 28, 38, 69, 72, 77, 78, 83, 84, 86, 88, 135, 141, 148, 151, 166, 168
transformation, 92, 93, 96, 97, 98, 99, 103, 110, 111
transition period, 294

transparency, ix, 29, 32, 65, 68, 88, 133, 140, 156, 212
transplant, 74
Treasury, 233
treatment, 92, 95, 97, 100, 145, 173, 194, 220, 234
tubal ligation, 146, 179
turnover, 180

U

U.S. economy, 34, 65, 69
underwriting, 242, 245, 246, 249, 253, 254, 255, 263, 264
uninsured, 179, 216, 217, 220, 222, 224, 229, 234, 235, 238, 241, 246, 247, 254, 259, 265, 270, 275, 281, 291
United States, 2, 6, 14, 15, 16, 17, 26, 33, 53, 73, 93, 102, 105, 122, 133, 134, 164, 166, 167, 183, 188, 198, 200, 226, 263, 283
universal access, 291
urban, 183, 253, 258
Urban Institute, 253, 258
USA, 285

V

vegetables, 269
venture capital, 103, 108, 109
vertical integration, 4, 7, 50, 80, 154, 167, 177, 197, 204, 205
vertical merger, 4, 7, 15, 17, 153, 165

vision, 111, 154
vote, 89, 122
voting, 260

W

wage increases, 36
wages, 36, 37, 118, 285, 287
walking, 285
Washington, 1, 30, 54, 55, 56, 58, 76, 189, 197, 199, 201, 209, 230, 249, 291, 295
waste, 113
water, 180, 215, 226
websites, 105
welfare, 146, 222, 223, 224, 284
well-being, 289
White House, 185
White Paper, 34
wholesale, 99
windows, 233
witnesses, 2, 5, 9, 11, 12, 13, 14, 18, 19, 25, 126, 139, 142, 145, 161, 210, 213, 274, 276, 281, 288
workers, 3, 6, 36, 118, 286
working class, 260
worry, 20, 145, 215, 236

Y

yield, 11, 14, 19, 22, 25, 81, 126, 129, 132, 139, 144, 148, 151, 153, 160, 213, 214, 261, 264, 269, 271, 274, 279, 281
young adults, 247

Related Nova Publications

IMPROVEMENTS NEEDED IN THE VA HEALTH CARE SYSTEM

EDITOR: Charles Copeland

SERIES: Health Care in Transition

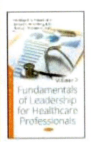

BOOK DESCRIPTION: Nearly 40,000 providers hold privileges in VHA's 170 VA Medical Centers (VAMCs). VAMCs must identify and review any concerns that arise about the clinical care their providers deliver.

HARDCOVER ISBN: 978-1-53615-971-4
RETAIL PRICE: $230

FUNDAMENTALS OF LEADERSHIP FOR HEALTHCARE PROFESSIONALS. VOLUME 2

EDITOR: Stanislaw P. A. Stawicki, MD, Michael S. Firstenberg, MD, and Thomas J. Papadimos, MD

SERIES: Health Care in Transition

BOOK DESCRIPTION: The current tome begins with an introductory chapter that provides an in-depth overview of various theoretical aspects of leadership, including the most commonly encountered leadership styles.

HARDCOVER ISBN: 978-1-53615-729-1
RETAIL PRICE: $230

To see a complete list of Nova publications, please visit our website at www.novapublishers.com

Related Nova Publications

GOVERNMENT REPORTS ON HEALTH CARE FOR MARCH 2019

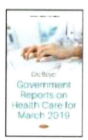

EDITOR: Eric Beyer

SERIES: Health Care in Transition

BOOK DESCRIPTION: This book is a comprehensive compilation of all reports, testimony, correspondence and other publications issued by the GAO (Government Accountability Office) during the month of March, grouped according to the topic: Health Care.

HARDCOVER ISBN: 978-1-53615-844-1
RETAIL PRICE: $160

To see a complete list of Nova publications, please visit our website at www.novapublishers.com